A Woman's Guide
to Martial Arts

A Woman's Guide to Martial Arts

How to Choose and Get Started in a Discipline

Monica McCabe Cardoza

THE OVERLOOK PRESS

WOODSTOCK • NEW YORK

First published in paperback in 1998 by
The Overlook Press, Peter Mayer Publishers, Inc.
Lewis Hollow Road
Woodstock, New York 12498

Library of Congress Cataloging-in-Publications Data

McCabe Cardoza, Monica.
A woman's guide to martial arts / Monica McCabe Cardoza.
p. cm.
1. Martial arts. 2. Self-defense for women. I. Title
GV1101.M33 1996 796.8—dc20 96-483

BOOK DESIGN AND FORMATTING BY BERNARD SCHLEIFER

Manufactured in the United States of America

First Edition

1 3 5 7 9 8 6 4 2

ISBN 0-87951-670-4 (hc)
ISBN 0-87951-843-X (pbk)

To David, Avery, and my parents.

Contents

Part I. Before Signing on the Dotted Line

1.
WHY THE MARTIAL ARTS?   17

Getting started in the martial arts will be tougher than any sparring match you're likely to encounter in your training. But the rewards are worth it.

Defining Excellence   19

Thriving and excelling in the martial arts doesn't mean rising through the ranks in record time.

Mind Over Matter   21

Strength is an asset, but conditioning the mind to plan and strategize moves is equally important.

The Key to Chi   23

Traceable to yoga, this ancient breathing technique rejuvenates the mind and strengthens the body.

Martial Arts Heroines   25

It was once as common for Asian women to learn to fight as it was to cook or pour tea—many of these women even went on to become powerful, well-respected warriors.

Why Some Train, Why Some Quit   29

A survey reveals what draws women to the martial arts, and what spurs some of them to leave.

Martial Myths   32

Competing in tournaments is mandatory. Sparring is an unpleasant fact of martial arts life.

On a More Personal Level   *136*

Strict rules on jewelry, hair clips, and nail care are zealously enforced because the injuries they can cause are highly preventable.

Protect Yourself   *140*

As your knowledge of the martial arts grows, so will your arsenal of protective equipment.

7.
BACK TO BASICS   *144*

The strong reliance on martial arts tradition coupled with the almost maniacal importance placed on performing basic moves over and over again lead to giant leaps in terms of self-discovery and self-improvement.

Stretching Your Limits   *146*

Flexibility is an essential element that sets the stage for maintaining interest and excelling in the martial arts. Here's how to safely and thoroughly stretch your muscles.

Strong–Arm Tactics   *153*

What you lack in physical strength can be compensated for in other areas.

Avoiding Injury   *157*

Yes, it's possible. Here's how.

Training Equipment   *160*

Punching pads and bags are the most common, but many schools also utilize updated versions of ancient training tools.

8.
LIFE IMITATES THE MARTIAL ARTS   *166*

Women's rise in the martial arts world is not dissimilar to the significant inroads they have made in the business world.

Opening Doors to Women   *168*

Desperate to keep their businesses afloat, martial arts instructors eagerly accepted female students, forcing male students to interact with females on unfamiliar, and often uncomfortable, levels.

Preface

After deciding to study a martial art, I found myself standing in the sports sections of several bookstores searching for a book that would tell me what I could expect, how to choose a reputable school and teacher, what styles best suited women, and how I could get the most out of my training—a book that would empower me to walk into a martial arts school with confidence and the right questions to ask the instructor.

I never found that book, so I decided to write it. With an undergraduate degree in journalism, a master's degree in publishing, and eight years of karate training under my belt, I spent three years researching and drawing on my own experiences. The result is *A Woman's Guide to Martial Arts,* an in-depth look into a sport that throughout history has proved ideal for women, and continues to draw women in increasing numbers.

A Woman's Guide to Martial Arts is a perfect first step for any woman wanting to get started in the martial arts. Beginning a new sport is never easy. But it is my hope that this book will strengthen your determination to pursue a martial art and that once you find your martial art niche, you remain committed and reap as much fulfillment as I have from this physically, mentally, and spiritually challenging sport.

MONICA MCCABE CARDOZA
Ridgewood, NJ 1996

Foreword

by Carol A. Wiley

After studying martial arts for 17 years, it's easy to forget the trepidation that new students often bring to their training. But when I look back at my early martial arts experience, I know how real the trepidation is. As a teenager, the martial arts attracted me, but I was shy, unathletic, and not particularly self-confident. It was my third attempt at taking a martial arts class before I stuck with it, some six years after my initial interest.

In my years of training I have seen more students come and go than I can possibly remember. People quit training for many reasons, but often the underlying cause is failure to understand the long-term nature of martial arts training. You do not learn a martial art in a few months—it is a pursuit where the learning never stops and where the only true measure of success comes from within. Perhaps the 17-year-old kid who started months after you does beautiful flying side kicks while you can barely get off the ground, but that's not important. What is important is that you are using your training to develop your skills.

To develop these skills, you must first get started. In *A Woman's Guide to the Martial Arts*, Monica McCabe Cardoza provides background information about many aspects of martial arts, especially those related to karate. The martial arts are so diverse that no book can possibly touch on all the possibilities you might encounter. But with the information in this book, you have a foundation on which you can build as you explore the martial arts world.

The best way to begin your exploration is to watch martial arts classes and talk to martial artists, both beginning and experienced. But, please, don't ask the dreaded question, "What is the best martial art?" Every martial art has its strengths and weaknesses, and any martial art is only as good as the practitioner.

Ask martial artists about their experiences. Ask why they study a particular martial art. Don't be surprised when you hear contradictory information—you'll find plenty of it. In the end, you'll have to go with what feels right for you. If your first choice doesn't work, try again. Don't let one bad experience turn you off to all the martial arts.

Probably one of the biggest controversies in the martial arts is that of traditional martial art versus sport martial art. Tournament competition is quite popular, but traditionalists argue that competition dilutes martial art techniques since only limited techniques can be used in tournament sparring without hurting one's opponent. If you understand that neither tournament technique nor traditional basic martial arts practice is street self-defense, you see the broad range of approaches you'll find in the martial arts world.

This world is still a male-dominated one, and being a woman in the martial arts is similar to being a woman in any other male-dominated field, with both challenges and rewards for those who persevere. Sometimes you have to work harder to be taken seriously. You may encounter pre-historic attitudes, and unfortunately sexual harassment is not unheard of. Sometimes you have to deal with subtle inequalities that men may not even be conscious of. Handle any issues that arise in a straight-forward, matter-of-fact manner, and you'll stay a step ahead.

More women are training than ever before, and more

women are reaching high ranks where they have an influence on the development of the martial arts. Some women run women-only martial arts schools. That's another controversy. Some people feel that training with women only doesn't provide the wide range of experience you would get training with men. But training in a women-only environment meets the needs of some women. You decide which is best for you.

Even if you elect to train in a mostly male environment, two organizations offer the opportunity to get together with other women and share information and experiences. The National Women Martial Arts Federation and the Pacific Association of Women Martial Artists both conduct annual training camps for women of all martial arts. Although I have always trained with men, attending these camps has been a refreshing and educational experience.

For most beginners, I believe the quality of the instructor is far more important than which art you choose. Some people are naturally drawn to a particular art, but if you aren't, concentrate on finding a top-quality instructor who emphasizes the aspects of the martial arts that most interest you. Having a top-quality tournament instructor is pointless if your main interest is self-defense. Also allow for the possibility that your interests will change. And once you choose a school and instructor, be willing to participate in what they offer. There's always something to learn.

Remember that even the best instructors are only human. Don't fall into the guru trap of thinking an instructor is infallible; you will only be disappointed. If an instructor or the other students promote this guru-type thinking, seriously consider moving on.

Instructors vary tremendously in what they expect from students and how they run their schools. Some schools have an almost military structure, while others are very laid back Some arts, for example traditional Japanese martial arts, are very formal and other arts, for example Brazilian Capoeira and the Filipino arts such as Arnis, are quite informal.

Getting the most from your martial arts training is your responsibility. Know your limits but don't be bound by them. The point of training is to learn and grow. Learn to push yourself but know when it's time to take a break, or, as I did, you may end up with your arm in a cast because of a stupid mistake.

During class, focus on your training and leave everything else at the door. Not only will you learn more, you will also help create a safer training environment—some of the worse accidents are the result of inattentiveness.

Be open to training with everyone, but if you encounter someone who is abusive, be willing to walk away. Be willing to ask your partner to train at a level you can handle. Learn to protect yourself in your training; even the best-intentioned partners make mistakes.

Protecting yourself also means taking care of your body. If some part of your body is weak (backs and knees are common problems), find what you need to do to strengthen these areas. For me, less than 10 minutes of knee exercises three or four times a week has been enough to get rid of the almost constant aching that had developed in my knees. Don't wait until something becomes a big problem—take care of it at the first signs of trouble.

Martial arts training requires a commitment. You can choose the level of commitment, but remember that you get out of something what you put into it. Find a level that suits your personality and life commitments. Whether you consider martial arts a hobby or find a deep passion for martial arts in your life, you will find the effects of training showing up in your life outside of class. Take your training and make the most of it—it's a commitment well worth making.

---

1. Why the Martial Arts?

GETTING STARTED in the martial arts was tougher than any sparring match I've since encountered in my eight years of training.

I chose a school, or "dojo," as martial artists refer to it, from the yellow pages, letting my fingers do the walking instead of my feet. My selection was based primarily on location. As a high school student without a driver's license, I chose a school close enough to my home that my father wouldn't be too inconvenienced dropping me off and picking me up from class three times a week. Fortunately, I chose a reputable school headed by an experienced teacher who taught an interesting form of traditional karate.

Two years and a green belt later, I stopped practicing karate when I went away to college. Though I did try the karate classes offered at college, they seemed too crowded and unfocused. It would be five years before I would return to the martial arts.

Working behind a desk for a couple of years made me quickly realize that I would either have to accept weight gain or fight it. So, returning to karate seemed a logical way to maintain a high-energy level and a small rear end. Having returned to the area in which I lived prior to college, I naturally decided to return to my original school. Unfortunately, it had moved to a location I considered too far away.

It was back to the yellow pages. This time, beyond location, I wanted a school that taught the same form of karate I had studied. That certainly narrowed down the choices. I subsequently found a school that was within walking distance to a stop on the train line I used to commute to my job in Manhattan. I could get off the train, grab my uniform from my car, and walk to class. On weekends, I could drive to the school in fifteen minutes. Of course, I didn't know it then, but that school, Budo Kai in River Edge, New Jersey, run under the auspices of Richard Rohrman, would see me through my black belt.

It all seemed perfect, except for the fact that I hadn't met the instructor or evaluated the school. At least I had enough of a background in the martial arts to know what questions to ask and how to observe a class. Such was not the case when I first joined a martial arts school. Back then I didn't know if the school would be receptive to women. I didn't know what questions to ask the teacher to find out; in fact, I wasn't sure I was allowed to ask him questions directly. Did he have assistants who screened questions like mine before passing them on to the teacher? How should the teacher be addressed? Sir? Master? Teacher? Mister? I remember, minutes away from starting my first class, fumbling as I tried to tie my belt, too intimidated to ask for help. Once on the floor, I realized I didn't know how to address students, or what other rules of etiquette applied on the training floor.

But what was perhaps most intimidating about starting in the martial arts was the proportion of men to women in my first school. Sprinkled throughout the class of twenty or so students were, at best, three females. What, I thought, could possibly be going through these women's minds? Did they feel as out of place as I did?

For the most part, no, they didn't. As I would soon discover, in properly run martial arts schools, gender doesn't play a significant role. Though the issue does come up even in the best schools, and some female martial artists report friction among themselves and male students, as a whole, the martial arts is a fairly nondiscriminatory sport. And, as I have discovered through my research for this book, many martial arts traditionally never distinguished between male and female. Understanding this basic, yet little known, aspect of the martial arts is one of the keys to thriving and excelling in them.

Defining Excellence

Thriving and excelling in the martial arts doesn't mean rising through the ranks in record time. The student who is promoted every six months may be no better than the student from the same class who is promoted every nine months, or once a year.

Maybe one student trains twice a week, while the other three or four times a week. Perhaps one student excels at sparring and self-defense techniques, while the other at forms and weapons. What's important is not that one student is promoted more often than another, but that both students are satisfied with their achievements.

Thriving and excelling in the martial arts means getting out of the sport what you want. Whether it's weight loss, self-discipline, flexibility, self-defense techniques, or tournament trophies—or all of the above—the purpose is to excel in what you want to excel in.

Too often, students become all-consumed with being promoted. Many often think, usually without justification, that the instructor has it out for them, and is holding them back. They compare themselves to other students, counting the days it took their contemporaries to earn their belts, then comparing it to the number of days they had to wait to receive the same colored belt.

If your goal is to tie a different-colored belt around your waist every three or four months, you may want to rethink the martial arts as the sport for you. Chances are you won't enjoy the training, and your classmates won't enjoy your company.

Of course, that's not to say that you may come to a point in your training when you believe you're due for a promotion. If that happens, take your case to the instructor, not other students. Differences of opinion are as common in martial arts schools as they are in the office and at home. As such, they're best dealt with calmly and directly.

MARTIAL MAXIM: EARNING A BLACK BELT MEANS NOTHING MORE THAN THAT THE STUDENT HAS MASTERED THE BASICS. NOW SHE IS READY TO LEARN AND GROW AS A MARTIAL ARTIST.

Those students who take up a martial art with the sole intent of earning a black belt in a short time, say a year or two—and I've met several—will likely drop out due to frustration at not being promoted as fast as they think they should be. Often they'll leave the school for another whose teacher promises the student a black belt in a set period of time.

In schools such as these, an instructor's desire to pass on the knowledge of a martial art to a student is often less important than the student's ability to pay tuition. (Though instructors aren't expected to carry students who can't or don't pay, teachers should at least have enough respect for their style of martial art to want to spend the time teaching it properly.) Gimmicks such as fast-tracks to black belts are seen by some instructors as incentives for students to stay with a school. True, these students eventually receive the black belt they are so intent on having—and they may even learn a thing or two.

But you can be sure they won't go around boasting to their friends about their shortcut to the top.

How can you spot such students? It's relatively easy. They're the ones who go out of their way to impress upon everyone within earshot their black-belt status. The martial arts to these individuals are trivialized to the status of a tool used to wield before astonished friends and acquaintances. That their black-belt contemporaries may have sweated more and trained longer is something they'd rather not discuss.

Serious, experienced martial artists don't use their skills to impress. They're the ones who never seem to talk about their training, unless someone asks about it or they're with some of their martial arts classmates. Their demeanor belies the fact that they study a martial art. Why? Their training is something they do for themselves, not for others.

True martial artists are a lot like artists in general. Whether a painter, sculptor, or writer, serious artists generally share an innate humbleness about themselves. As artists, they know that no matter what any one person's opinion, they first have to believe in themselves.

Mind Over Matter

Certainly, the martial arts is an introspective sport. Just about everyone is familiar with the stereotype of the quiet, shy martial artist who when provoked explodes in a fury of kicks and punches, leaving the oversized, muscular assailant a dusty heap on the floor.

While this overused scene has by now become almost cliché, there is an aspect of it that is readily apparent: the inner strength that seems to emanate from the martial artist. In Japan, this trait is known as ki and is pronounced KEE. In China, it is called chi and is pronounced CHEE.

Chi is an energy that is cultivated by the mind. One reason women are well-suited to the martial arts is that what they lack in strength, they can more than make up for in mental ability. This ability to think, or use the mind to control the body, is another key to succeeding in the martial arts.

Some veteran martial artists report that they can feel their chi, describing it as an energy that passes through their lower abdomen. Others pinpoint it to an inch below the navel, which is thought to be the center, or most balanced point, of a person. But feeling chi is a long way from being able to control it.

MARTIAL MAXIM: THERE IS AN ENERGY WITHIN EVERYONE THAT THE MARTIAL ARTS CULTIVATES THROUGH CONCENTRATION AND BREATHING EXERCISES.

This mastery doesn't come overnight. In fact, it can take a lifetime to achieve. Those who can control their chi—and they are few and far between—often exhibit unusual powers. One aikido master can supposedly use his chi to plant himself into the floor, immune to anyone who tries to move him. Other chi masters can throw an attacker with a simple touch of their hand.

But chi isn't selective. It's in everyone. You've heard about the mother who knocks down a heavy door because her child is locked in a burning room. Or the husband who lifts a car because his wife's leg is pinned beneath. The difference between these individuals and a master of chi lies in the situations. In an emergency, people act almost without thinking, only later fully comprehending the enormity of the feat they've accomplished. A martial artist is taught to pinpoint and cultivate this strength in order to draw on it at anytime.

But don't be too concerned with controlling your chi. What's important is not controlling it, but being aware of it, knowing it's in you, then using that knowledge to further yourself as a martial arts student and as a human being. As you begin training, you might be called on to perform a kata in front of the class. (A kata is simply a series of attacking and blocking techniques strung together. Katas were choreographed by martial arts masters to allow students to practice self-defense techniques on their own.) Drawing on your chi will allow you to put aside your apprehension or intimidation and perform to the best of your ability. Even outside your school, you'll recognize your chi and draw on it when you need that extra boost of confidence.

As your training sessions become progressively harder, you may find yourself calling on your chi to get through a tough workout. By drawing on chi, you'll find the mental strength to tell your body to do another kick or punch—and maybe even another after that. In fact, you'll surprise yourself at just how much you can do if you, literally, put your mind to it.

The Key to Chi

Chi isn't something martial artists discovered. It can be traced to the gentle art of yoga—certainly an art in which women have long been active participants. In fact, when people talk about the martial arts as a gentle art, they are in part referring to its roots in yoga and meditation.

In yoga, chi passes through the "hara," or stomach. One way practitioners of yoga and the martial arts cultivate this energy is through controlled breathing techniques. In the martial arts, controlled breathing plays an important role as a meditative exercise performed before and after class in order to clear the mind of the day's worries and to improve concentration. During class, breathing is stressed as a way to keep students energetic.

How many times have you heard an aerobics instructor

remind new students to keep breathing? If you've taken aerobics classes, chances are you've heard it a lot. You'll hear the same reminders in martial arts schools. Martial arts instructors must not only constantly tell new students to keep breathing, but to breathe properly—taking in air through the nose, then exhaling through the mouth.

When new students breathe properly, an almost mystical transformation takes place. Their shoulders drop to a comfortable, more natural position, their timing improves, and their stamina increases. Even their movements become cleaner and more reflexive because they are no longer thinking solely about what they're doing, but allowing it to become second nature.

> **MARTIAL MAXIM: IN LEARNING TO BREATHE PROPERLY, YOU'LL BE CALLED ON TO UTILIZE YOUR DIAPHRAGM, AN ORGAN THAT INFANTS AND SMALL CHILDREN USE EXCLUSIVELY FOR BREATHING.**

To alleviate anxiety before class, and to wind down after class, many martial arts teachers have students sit on the floor and perform a yoga-related breathing exercise that utilizes the diaphragm. Here, the diaphragm—which separates the chest from the abdominal cavities—pushes the abdominal organs down and forward, rhythmically and gently massaging and compressing the abdominal organs. Instead of your ribs expanding when you inhale, your stomach protrudes as it fills with air.

To most new students, stomach breathing feels unnatural and uncomfortable, while breathing that expands the chest area feels natural. With all the pressure to have a flat stomach, it's no wonder. However, as you practice it and integrate it into your workouts, diaphragmatic breathing will become more natural. What's more, you'll find that, physiologically, it is more efficient and relaxing.

By now, you may be noticing that the martial arts are aptly named. Just as true martial artists have an innate humbleness about them, like many artists in general, learning to breathe properly is in itself an art. This will become more apparent as you continue training. You'll not only come to appreciate the muscular strength you'll gain, but you'll sense an equally powerful strength inside you. Indeed, the spiritual and artistic traits inherent in the martial arts are as powerful and potent a force as the fighting techniques themselves.

Martial Arts Heroines

Adding to the spirituality of the martial arts through the influences of yoga, chi, and meditation is the enormous role that religious leaders played in the development of the arts. Adding to the nondiscriminatory nature of the arts is the influential role women played in the arts' formative years.

During the fifth and sixth centuries, Zen Buddhist monks and nuns brought from India to China yoga and Indian fist-fighting techniques similar to modern karate. These fighting techniques came in handy in war-torn China. Indeed, learning to fight was as common as learning to cook or pour tea. Survival for men, women, and even children hinged on their ability to protect themselves. Those who excelled became notable warriors.

Thirteen-year-old Shuen Guan is a perfect example. Her ability to fight with swords, spears, and even her bare hands earned her the nickname "Little Tigress." According to one legend, she saved her town from an attack by bandits by fighting her way through the attackers and returning with a neighboring general and his troops. Her heroic deeds were eventually honored by the emperor of China.

But not everyone could be as multitalented as Shuen Guan. Specialization had a definite place in war-torn China. After learning a basic fighting skill, the tendency was to add moves and techniques to suit a particular ability or body type. For one woman named Ng Mui that meant redirecting her punches from the midsection of an attacker to the head, and throwing kicks to the lower legs.

Specialization enabled people to become masters of their own styles. Mui was so proficient at her style that to prove its effectiveness, she demonstrated her moves on martial arts masters themselves, who quickly came to realize that her methods would work as well for them as they did for her.

That Mui was a woman is impressive enough. But what makes her extraordinary to martial arts students who practice her style today is the fact that she was a Buddhist nun! She came from a Shaolin monastery in southern China during the Ching Dynasty.

One of Ng Mui's students, Yim Wing Chun, carried on this style after Mui's death. Eventually, this system became known as Wing Chun kung fu.

Interestingly, though developed for a woman, Wing Chun kung fu became the style of choice among many men. In fact, this style of kung fu grew stronger in popularity as the centuries rolled by, and became the preferred style of the late martial artist-turned-actor Bruce Lee, who introduced and popularized this style in the West in the 1960s and '70s. For those too young to remember, visit any video store where you'll find a wide selection of Bruce Lee movies. Though as grade B as a movie can get, they're worthwhile watching just to observe Lee's extraordinary athletic abilities.

Judo, too, has some distinctly female roots. While kung fu grew out of China, judo has its roots in the fighting systems of feudal Japan, which from the tenth to the eighteenth centuries found itself awash in samurais—highly skilled fighters who, often on horseback, battled with bows and arrows, swords, and spears.

In the early part of this period, samurai women shared the

battlefield with men—and occasionally commanded them. These martial matriarchs were often trained in the use of weapons, especially spears and small daggers.

One of the favored weapons among samurai on horseback was the naginata, a long pole, from five to nine feet, with a sword at the end. Occasionally called "the woman's spear," the naginata was the weapon of choice for Itagaki, a female general in charge of three-thousand warriors in 1199. Her expertise and courage supposedly inspired her troops and shamed the enemy.

Another famous woman warrior of the same period was Tomoe. The name means "circular" or "turning," and was probably given to her because of her mastery of the naginata, which is used by making circular movements.

Woman warriors continued to fight up until one of the last civil wars in Japan. In 1877, a battle was fought with a group of 500 women in its ranks. These women, armed with naginatas, fought against Japanese government troops. Unfortunately, their skills were no match against the guns carried by their opponents.

If you were lucky enough to be a female born into a ninja family, chances are you would be taught, along with your brother if you had one, starting at the age of five or six, to be a superior athlete. By the age of twelve or thirteen, you might move on to weapons training.

Ninja were latter-day James Bonds: superagents who were not only superior fighters, but masters at disguise. Men often dressed as women, and vice versa.

In the mid- to late 1800s, as there became less of a need for samurai, women's influence in the martial arts declined. Unless women came from a military family, it was considered scandalous for them to train alongside men in martial arts schools. If any training went on, it was done in private.

Scandalous or not, many women wanted to practice a

martial art, and did. In 1893, Sueko Ashiya became the first women student of Jigoro Kano, who founded judo in Japan. Soon after he took on Ashiya, Kano began teaching his wife, daughter, and their female friends.

In the mid-1920s, Kano opened a women's section of his school so his female students could train in a proper environment. Though a major breakthrough that guaranteed many women the opportunity to train, Japanese women today still train only in the women's section, and except for special situations are not allowed to train with men.

MARTIAL MAXIM: WOMEN HAVE NOT YET REGAINED THEIR EQUAL STATUS IN THE MARTIAL ARTS. BUT THEY'RE CLOSER TODAY THAN THEY WERE SEVERAL YEARS AGO.

But don't think that old habits die hard only in the Orient. Up until about 1976, the belts worn by female judo martial artists had to have a white stripe running down the middle if the women wanted to compete in national competitions. The ruling was changed, however, thanks to a few determined women who demonstrated their disapproval of the rule by fighting in competitions wearing only white belts, refusing to wear a colored belt with a stripe in it.

Consider another rule that prevented women from achieving the same rank as men. Kano's original school prohibited black belt women from being promoted higher than fifth dan, while men could go as high as twelfth dan. In 1972 the school received letters from women all over the world protesting this rule and asking the school to promote one of its leading female students, Keiko Fukuda, who had received her fifth-degree black belt in 1953. The letter-writing campaign worked, and Fukuda became the first woman sixth dan in the world—almost twenty years after becoming a fifth dan.

Karate also never traditionally distinguished between male

and female. Karate originated in Okinawa as a defense against Japanese invaders who stripped the natives of their weapons. In addition to using their hands and feet, Okinawans utilized farm tools to attack their oppressors. Women and men would practice their skills alone in the forests or fields using sickles or bamboo polls. Eventually, even a harmless-looking farm woman reaping her crops became a force to contend with.

Sport karate became increasingly popular and widespread in the 1940s. While competition was originally limited primarily to men, women now compete in both sparring and kata tournaments. There are even some mixed forms competitions, and occasionally mixed sparring between men and women.

Today, notable female martial artists can be found in every style of martial art—from kick boxer Kathy Long to karate champion Cynthia Rothrock. These women, and others like them, are the modern-day equivalents of the women warriors of centuries ago. Their determination to carve a niche for themselves in this sport is a shining example to every female martial artist.

Why Some Train, Why Some Quit

Why are women drawn to the martial arts? A survey in *Black Belt* magazine sought to answer that question. The findings may help you prioritize the reasons why you want to study a martial art.

The *Black Belt* survey incorporates the responses of forty female martial artists, ranging in age from seven to sixty, and ranging in rank from white to black belt. It encompasses several different martial arts styles and covers women with more than twenty-five years of training to women who have dropped out of the martial arts.

Most of the women (38 percent) began training for self-defense reasons. Some were victims of rape or battery, and some feared physical retribution because of a legal matter such as a divorce.

That most women took up a martial art for self-defense reasons is a sad reflection on society. However, the unfortunate reality remains that no woman is immune to violence—whether it happens while shopping in a mall, attending school, working in an office, taking a walk, or just being home, and whether it's by a stranger or a former or current boyfriend or spouse. This sad fact of modern-day life has sent thousands of women running to sign up for basic, no-frills self-defense courses. Never mind spirituality or proper form, these women want to learn fast, quick methods to ward off attackers.

Such demand has given rise to numerous so-called assault-prevention schools. From Model Mugging of Boston Inc. to Impact Personal Safety of Van Nuys, California, to Out of Harm's Way Inc. of Etobicoke, Ontario, these schools re-create assaults, often using well-padded male "attackers," to teach women how to protect themselves. In some cases, employers pick up the tab for their employees to attend these classes, and even allow the classes to take place at the office.

Does this spell the demise of the martial arts? Certainly not. While the martial arts teaches self-defense techniques, it takes years of training to be able to apply those moves on the street. The prevalence of assault-prevention schools simply means that women will have more choices and those who want only to learn self-defense will seek out these facilities.

For many women, self-defense is simply an added benefit of martial arts training. What they really like about the martial arts is the challenge it presents—something missing from their current workouts. And the *Black Belt* survey results bear this out.

MARTIAL MAXIM: IF ALL YOU'RE SEEKING IS SELF-DEFENSE INSTRUCTION, TRY ONE OF THE NEW "ASSAULT-PREVENTION" SCHOOLS THAT HAVE RECENTLY CROPPED UP.

According to the survey, 22 percent of the women found martial arts more physically and mentally challenging than other sports. To that extent, it gave the women the aerobic conditioning of running or jazzercize—minus the boredom—with the added benefits of self-confidence, self-defense, and improved discipline.

Indeed, more women today seem to be intentionally seeking out sports that involve a great deal more risk than conventional workouts such as aerobics. Thanks to these women, today's female sports figures are portrayed more as heroines than as oddities, which up until a few decades ago would have been the norm. Certainly, the image of the female athlete has changed a great deal. Whereas the image of a makeup-free, sweaty woman resting after a long, hard workout would have been considered unappealing several years ago, today manufacturers such as Nike and Reebok use this image widely in their ads, presenting athleticism as female autonomy, self-mastery, self-expression, and individuality. Naomi Wolf, author of *The Beauty Myth* (Doubleday, 1991) and *Fire With Fire* (Random House, 1993), put it succinctly in a 1994 interview for *Women's Sports & Fitness* magazine: "Sports gives women the sense that their bodies belong to them," she said.

One-quarter of the women who participated in the *Black Belt* survey joined a martial arts school because a family member or friend was already enrolled and enjoyed the training. One women signed up for classes because she was tired of spending weekends while her husband competed at tournaments, today she competes in tournaments, too. The remaining 15 percent of the women joined because the training looked interesting or fun, for aesthetic reasons such as the grace and fluidity of the forms, to add discipline to their lives, or to reduce stress.

The fact that a martial arts magazine surveyed women is an enormous step in the right direction. Certainly, when I started training eight years ago, few in the field were interested in what women thought. But competition among the numerous martial arts schools, coupled with the recession of the early '90s, has forced instructors to pay more attention to their female students, both those they have and those they could have.

Use this situation to your advantage. Tell your instructor what you want out of your training. Two years ago, your requests might have fallen on deaf ears. Today, chances are that your suggestions will be taken seriously—and if they're not, the school may not be right for you. Besides, if you think something is missing from your martial arts training program, chances are some of your classmates feel the same way.

Martial Myths

While the *Black Belt* survey results point out the reasons women take up a martial art, they don't reveal why some respondents dropped out, or why some women, though drawn to the sport, never pursue it. Interestingly, among the women I've spoken with—women who were intrigued by the martial arts, but never pursued one of them—several have indicated some very specific reasons why they would not study a martial art. Their reasons point to common fallacies surrounding the arts, which I call "martial arts myths."

Martial arts myths aren't usually started by individuals outside the martial arts. They are often perpetuated by the very people who study them. Only when one studies a martial art does the realization surface that these myths are just that—myths!

Well, it's time to put to rest some of the misconceptions surrounding the martial arts. Let's start with the more blatant ones. As you continue reading this book, you'll discover other myths that will surprise you.

• Competing in tournaments is mandatory. In all my years of training, I participated in just one tournament. Though I had no desire to compete, when a group of my karate classmates invited me to join them at a tournament being held at a nearby university, I decided the experience would be beneficial.

With sparring ranking down there with push-ups on my scale of most-enjoyable martial arts activities, I decided to forgo sparring competition and signed up with other green belts in kata competition, in which students perform pre-arranged movements incorporating various techniques. I must have done fairly well because I took third place. However, the experience didn't thrill me as it did some of my contemporaries who enjoyed performing before an audience and competing for awards and recognition.

The fact that I would never compete again did not in any way hold me back or slow me down from rising through the martial arts ranks. Competing is something you do for yourself, and if your instructor insists that you compete, my advice is to find another one.

• Sparring is an unpleasant fact of martial arts life. Most schools require their students to spar. But if you remember from the *Black Belt* survey, no women took up a martial art to spar. In fact, among women, sparring is one of the toughest aspects of their training.

A good instructor understands new students' apprehension regarding sparring and consequently eases them into it, first by letting the students simply observe other students spar, then allowing the new students to spar slowly and lightly with high-ranking students. Later, new students will step up the pace and spar with a wider range of students.

If properly initiated into sparring, students will not only learn to enjoy it, but excel at it as well. Remember, sparring is a give-and-take exercise. When sparring partners understand this, they are far more likely to sustain fewer injuries.

I accumulated more injuries and angry emotions sparring as a middle-ranking green belt than as a beginner white belt or as an advanced black belt. As a green belt, I was expected to spar as hard and fast as high-ranking students. No longer protected like I was as a white belt, and trying to prove that I was brown-belt material, I took more risks and was apt to make more poor judgments than at any other time in my training.

(In my training, new students start as white belts, progressing to yellow, green, brown, then the high-ranking black belt. In between each color, students receive "tabs," which in my school are nothing more than colored electrical tape that is wrapped around each end of the belt and signify that the student is progressing to her next colored belt. Other schools may use different colored belts, including orange and purple, but most schools rank black-belt students similarly, with these students progressing from the beginning first-degree black belt to tenth-degree black belt, the highest rank achieved only by a few.)

By the time I earned my black belt, I had learned that sparring is something you do at your own pace. Unfortunately, this realization came late in the game. But the same needn't happen to you. Don't let anxiety or aggressive surges overcome you during a sparring session. And especially don't feel pressured to throw multiple kicks and punches at your opponent. If you throw even one clean strong kick or punch during a sparring match, you've accomplished a lot.

- Instructors are obsessed with perfection. We should all

strive for perfection. But when an instructor pushes students to the point at which they're uncomfortable and unhappy, then perhaps the instructor has gone too far. If you find yourself in this situation, discuss it in private with your instructor. Just because the martial arts require seriousness and determination doesn't mean you can't laugh a little and enjoy your training.

• Humiliation is part of the curriculum. The rule here is simple: No one deserves to be humiliated. If your instructor does or says something that embarrasses you, tell him or her in private that it bothered you. If it happens again, find another school.

• Breaking wooden boards with the blow of a bare hand is the sign of an experienced martial artist. It's not unusual to attend tournaments during which martial artists break boards with their hands, feet, or heads. The practice continues despite the fact that some in the martial arts community deplore this display, often because it has more to do with hitting the board in just the right spot than with athletic ability.

My first karate instructor took a novel approach to this practice. He allowed his students to use their hands to break boards as well as a brick. (Actually, the "brick" had three large holes in it and was wrapped in a towel, and the instructor positioned it at such an angle that breaking it required relatively little strength or expertise.) After we each smashed through several wooden boards and then a brick, we realized that the act involved more showmanship than ability, and never took it seriously again.

• All martial arts are inherently violent. The martial arts do indeed instruct their practitioners to execute some very violent moves. But the fact remains that these arts also teach their disciples to react to violence, not provoke it. This basic truth is evident in martial arts students themselves who, as you'll discover throughout your training, are for the most part not only nonviolent, but antiviolent as well.

Five Keys for Succeeding in the Martial Arts

1. Thriving and excelling in the martial arts doesn't mean rising through the ranks in record time; thriving and excelling in the martial arts means getting out of the sport what you want.

2. By taking up a martial art, you are accepting new risks, both physical and mental. But more women are concluding that the self-esteem and power that come from facing these risks are well worth the challenge.

3. Those students who take up a martial art with the sole intent of earning a black belt in a short time are likely to drop out due to frustration at not being promoted as fast as they think they should be.

4. In the martial arts, breathing properly—taking in air through the nose, then exhaling through the mouth—is as important as any other part of your training, including forming a fist.

5. One reason women are well-suited to the martial arts is that what they lack in strength, they can more than make up for in mental ability. This ability to think, or use the mind to control the body, is key to succeeding in the martial arts.

2. Choosing the Right Style

YOU'VE MADE THE DECISION to try a martial art. Now comes the really tough part: Choosing a style.

Taking the time to evaluate the various styles of martial arts can mean the difference between enjoying your training and dreading it. Enjoying your martial arts training means you'll look forward to attending class, no one will have to prod you to go, and you'll arrive there anticipating a productive workout. By attending regularly, you'll feel more a part of the class, and you'll feel your moves improving as you sail smoothly through the workouts.

Dreading your training means you'll make excuse after excuse for not attending class, and when you run out of excuses, you'll drive to class in a near panic, fearing that your lack of attendance will show through during class. Once you get there, you may view your fellow classmates more as strangers than as partners, and the workouts may feel harder than they actually are, as you huff and puff your way through basic warm-ups.

Dreading your training may mean you chose the wrong style. Maybe it's too hard for you, or perhaps it involves too much grappling than you care for. Maybe you would have been better off following your own intuition instead of joining a school because a friend talked you into it. Or perhaps you should have done some research before investing your time and money in that school.

Certainly, doing even a small amount of research can make a big difference in your martial arts training. And research doesn't have to mean spending huge chunks of time at the library. Research also doesn't require buying every martial arts book ever published. It can be done selectively and (*see* Bibliography) inexpensively. But it does require a commitment, which you'll find is well worth it.

Researching the right martial arts style for you is important if only because there are hundreds of styles from which to choose. What's more, most schools do not teach the same style in the same way. But before you begin evaluating these types of differences, you need to have an understanding of the basic styles that form the foundation of all martial arts styles. This chapter will describe nine basic styles that are readily recognized by most people and that are likely to be taught in your neighborhood. They are:

- aikido
- judo
- karate
- kung fu
- tae kwon do
- tai chi chuan
- hapkido
- jujitsu
- kendo

Within some of the above-mentioned styles are substyles, which this chapter will also describe. For example, within aikido are some fourteen different styles. We'll describe three of them—the other eleven are not commonly found in today's schools.

Certainly, don't be put off by the hundreds of different

martial arts styles. As you read this chapter, it will become clear that in many cases, martial arts styles share more common traits than uncommon ones. One style may trace its roots to Korea and another to China, but both may incorporate the same energetic, powerful kicks. After all, a kick is a kick, and a punch is a punch. Whether the kick is thrown with one foot on the ground or both feet in the air is really just a minor difference. But it may make a big difference to you if, like me, your feet were never meant to leave the floor.

Different Styles, Similar Benefits

Regardless of the style you ultimately choose, you're likely to reap similar physical and mental benefits. For women, practicing a martial art taps the inherent strength in their legs and builds the upper body. In fact, when I started training, I was a size eight above my waist and a size ten below. Today, those numbers are reversed thanks to my training. Even my posture has improved.

As an added benefit to physical conditioning, the meditative aspects of my training produced a profound attitude change. I went from being shy to being self-confident; from impatient to patient; and from thinking things should be done one way to understanding that there's more than one way to accomplish the same goal.

As for workouts, even less aggressive styles provide their practitioners with training sessions that are as equally invigorating as an aerobics class. Just because many aikido and judo techniques are performed while standing in one place doesn't mean you won't get winded. The effort you'll expend on just rising from the mat every time you take a throw is itself a workout.

As you read about the different martial arts styles, think about choosing one that coincides with your personality and physical abilities. Don't join a school because it offers a popular style. For instance, much press, especially in women's magazines, has recently been given to a new breed of athletic actresses who have taken up kick boxing. These articles are quick to point out that women have strong leg muscles and are therefore prime candidates for this sport. However, the articles often fail to inform readers that it's a particularly rough sport, one that focuses almost exclusively on fighting.

In addition to matching your abilities to a particular martial arts style, think about why you want to study. Is it for self-defense reasons? Health reasons? Do you like how martial arts students look when they perform? Perhaps you're drawn to sports that emphasize mental abilities as well as physical abilities. Maybe it's all four reasons.

MARTIAL MAXIM: IF YOU'RE STUDYING A MARTIAL ART FOR FITNESS REASONS, BE SURE THE STYLE YOU CHOOSE SUITS YOUR PHYSICAL ABILITIES AND YOUR CONDITIONING GOALS.

Different styles tend to favor some parts of the body over others. That's why it's important to consider your strengths and weaknesses, and compare them to your favorite styles. Get a checkup and ask your doctor if your body, especially your knees, ankles, and lower back, can withstand an hour or more of strenuous exercise. My martial arts training actually strengthened my lower back, but it took its toll on my knees, which tend to click and lock if I don't thoroughly warm them up prior to a workout.

But keep in mind that you shouldn't dismiss a style just because it doesn't completely match your physical abilities. Schools compete so vigorously for students today that instructors will often tailor a martial arts program to avoid putting stress on a student's weak points. If you prefer a style that happens to use the knees a lot, and your knees aren't in great shape, don't assume you can't study that style. Discuss your concerns with the teacher, and be up-front, explaining that you like the style and his manner of teaching but may not physically be able to keep up with the class during every workout. A good teacher will try to work something out. Perhaps he will allow you to do sit-ups when the rest of the class performs deep knee bends, or to raise your stances so as not to stress the knees.

Too often new students continue exercising a weak joint, and quietly suffer the consequences. This not only stresses the joint, but lowers the student's morale. Don't be a martyr. Even if you have to be the first student to set a precedent in your school, do it! If you tell your instructor that you want to train hard, but need to avoid further damage to a weak area, your instructor will understand. (If he doesn't, find another one.) Taking this bold but necessary step will earn you the respect of your classmates, and will probably spur them to demand the same treatment for themselves.

Finally, be wary of any instructor who tells you one martial art is the better than another. Certainly, it's okay for an instructor to be partial to a particular style, but he shouldn't rule all others out except for the one he teaches. Remember, there is no martial art that's best suited to women. The best martial art is the one your body feels comfortable with, gives you self-confidence, and keeps you coming back for more.

How Many Schools Are There?

It's almost impossible to determine how many students participate in a particular martial art, or the number of schools that teach a particular style. The associations that represent each style—the United States Judo Federation, U.S.A. Karate Federation, U.S. Tae kwon do Union, World Martial Arts

Association, to name just a few—can only account for those schools that register with them. In some cases, there are triple the number of schools and students scattered throughout the country.

Keep in mind, too, that though martial arts styles share common characteristics, not even styles with the same name are similar. For example, the style of karate I study, Goju-ryu, probably differs from the Goju-ryu karate taught in other schools. My teacher's knowledge of this style is influenced by his past training as well as his interest in other martial arts styles. This is not unusual.

Historically, the tendency has been for students to master a martial art in the Orient, then introduce it in a foreign country where they more often than not redefined it—adding new moves, disregarding others, and refocusing the philosophy. Eventually, an essentially Western approach developed, one that focused on the needs of Western students and the need for the instructor to feel in control of "his" style.

Even instructors who try to adhere to the historically correct version of their style may find it difficult. Historical accounts are only as accurate as their authors wanted them to be. In ancient China, for example, it was not unusual for a school to keep secret its fighting techniques, or to pad the facts with various inaccuracies in order to confuse outsiders. Add to this the fact that many of the secrets were passed down through word of mouth, and you have a recipe for confusion.

The result of all this is a hodgepodge of styles that fall under a general category of, say, karate or kung fu. You'll realize this more when you begin talking to martial arts students—an important part of your research. Tell them you're interested in studying karate, and they're likely to ask, "What style of karate?" Understanding that there are substyles within karate will not only make you look knowledgeable, but may spur students to take a real interest in helping you find your martial arts niche. Note, too, that not-so-subtle differences probably exist among students who study the same substyle but at different schools. Who knows? Maybe after years of your own training, you'll open a school that teaches your own interpretation of your instructor's style.

As more Western martial artists develop their own styles, the line between Western and Eastern philosophy will continue to blur. Sure, some styles will continue to try to remain true to their martial arts roots, as their followers dedicate themselves to teaching the style as it was taught by its founder. At the other end of the spectrum are those who throw tradition to the wind. For example, one new style, developed by a martial artist/Hollywood fight scene choreographer, combines kung fu, karate, and judo, but eschews ceremony. Students don't bow, wear martial arts uniforms, learn Eastern terminology, or the history of their style. Instead, they wear sweats and sneakers and are more informal with their instructor. Is either way better? Probably not. It's what suits you best.

Nine Basic Styles

Following are descriptions of popular martial arts styles. Within each style are references to offshoot styles, as well as explanations of each style's philosophy, distinguishing characteristics, and the basic training techniques beginners are likely to encounter.

Remember that because martial arts styles are more similar than dissimilar, observing—not just reading about—them is the best way to decide which one is right for you. But for now, a basic primer on the various styles will help you before you observe classes. (Chapter 3 will describe how to observe a martial arts class.)

As you read through the different styles, you may notice that unlike most martial arts books, this one doesn't contain much Japanese, Korean, or Chinese terminology. This is done intentionally to avoid confusion and to make the reading more enjoyable. If you decide to pursue a martial art, you'll learn the appropriate terms soon enough. Also omitted are advanced moves that students who have trained for a long time typically learn. Again, you'll learn these techniques at the appropriate time.

•*Aikido*

Aikido is a relatively new martial art, invented in the 1930s by Morihei Ueshiba, a religious man who followed Shinto, the national religion of Japan. Roughly translated from Japanese, aikido means the "way of connecting with life energy." Behind this art is the belief that within each individual lies the possibility of power.

The Art of Throwing

As one of the softest of the soft styles of martial arts, aikido is easily recognizable by its circular, flowing movements that lead to a throw or a lock. Indeed, from a technical point of view, aikido is a throwing art. Unlike judo students, aikidoists don't grip their opponent's clothing, but either "push-strike" the opponent's body, or grip the opponent's hand or arm.

Unlike karate, aikido emphasizes throwing and joint techniques over striking and kicking techniques. It also requires that students take hard falls on a mat, and develop strong, flexible wrists and strong forearms.

The principle behind aikido involves blending with an opponent's energy and leading her from a common center. An aikido student applies force to her opponent's pressure points, as well as grappling techniques that turn the opponent's momentum against her. Interestingly, that force doesn't come from the student; it comes from the opponent. An aikido student uses her opponent's force by bringing it into her own circle, neutralizing it, then gaining control.

The concept of the circle plays a central role in aikido. Even when the attack is linear—an opponent charges you in a straight line—you grab your opponent, create a centrifugal force that neutralizes your opponent's momentum, then complete the throw. After training for a while, this free-flowing motion becomes second nature, and, when done well, produces an art that is both useful and aesthetically appealing.

As you can see, aikido is a defensive art—your focus is on defending yourself, not attacking, which is referred to as *offensive.* Though it does emphasize principles of nonconflict, it does so in such a way that once an aikidoist decides to react, she can send an attacker hurtling to the mat.

FALLING AND SLAPPING OUT

New aikido students learn to fall safely. This involves slapping the mat with the forearm and hand before the body hits the mat. It also involves learning how to roll by tucking in the head, rolling along the arm and shoulders, then slapping out with the other arm.

Then simple throwing, stepping, and locking techniques are taught from standing and sitting positions. Stepping techniques involve grabbing the wrist and learning to move in a direction that causes the opponent to drop to the mat. Eventually, you'll learn to throw your opponent from this grab. Variations on the wrist grab include using the free hand to lock the opponent by applying pressure just below her elbow.

Teaching students the concept of the circle often begins with demonstrations. For example, the teacher may instruct a student to charge a more advanced student, who grabs the charging student's wrist, guides her to a point where both their arms are extended, then, using the built-up centrifugal force, pulling their arms in the opposite direction, causing her opponent to fall onto the mat.

One of the first things you're likely to notice during these demonstrations is the almost effortless moves the advance student makes. Not only does she hardly move from her position, but her techniques have a distinct rhythm to them. Mastering techniques to this extent takes years of practice and a high degree of physical conditioning.

THREE POPULAR STYLES

Aikido incorporates some fourteen different styles; three of them that remain popular today were developed by Ueshiba's students—Kenji Tomiki, Koichi Tohei, and Gozo Shioda— and in two cases are named after them. Tomiki aikido is distinguished by its practical elements of self-defense, which is why it is often practiced competitively.

As in many martial arts styles, students can choose from several types of competition. In aikido they can compete in forms, which are prearranged movements, performed individually or in pairs, incorporating various techniques. They can compete in trios in a "free style" format in which techniques are performed randomly, and they can compete against one another using knives or short swords. Finally, they can compete in pairs, unarmed, by applying techniques.

At the other end of the aikido spectrum is Tohei aikido, which emphasizes the spirituality of the art, especially the concept of ki. In this style, the student's goal is to harmonize her ki with that of her opponent.

Yoshin aikido, founded by Shioda, is combat-oriented

though it doesn't advocate competition. It places less emphasis on ki, and more emphasis on "hard" training methods. The style incorporates some 150 basic techniques, which enable the student to master the remaining ones, which total some 3,000.

•Judo

Translated from the Japanese as the "gentle way," judo was developed as an educational tool. Its founder, Jigoro Kano, hoped that it would become the sport of Japan, and instill moral principles and physical well-being in the country's inhabitants. Borrowing what he knew from his jujitsu studies, Kano worked out his own theory that by giving in to the force of your opponent, you can turn that force to your advantage.

UNDER PRESSURE

Judo is a defensive art that teaches its practitioners to apply force to an opponent's pressure points—nerve centers located, for example, behind the jawbone, inside the armpit, and atop the collarbone, and which, when held properly, cause an opponent temporary pain or paralysis. Once this force is applied, the student uses grappling to turn the opponent's momentum against her.

Blows are delivered with a sharp recoiling action to different areas of the body using the fingertips, fist, elbows, edge of the hand, knees, ball of the foot, and the heel. Strikes are delivered to the bridge of the nose, temple, ear, upper lip, windpipe, solar plexus, kidney, groin, and knees. Soft grappling techniques are combined with hard foot sweeps to throw an opponent to the ground.

Some compare judo competitions to wrestling matches. And, indeed, judo has become a more competitive-oriented martial art that occasionally forgoes technique in order to win. However, there are still noncompetitive elements of Kano's judo that are widely practiced, including throwing techniques, breakfalling, and joint locking.

LEARNING TO FALL

One of the first things you're likely to learn in judo is how to fall—something you'll be doing a lot of, and in all directions. You'll learn to fall to the right and left sides, as well as backward and forward.

As in aikido, when you fall to the mat or are thrown, you must either break your fall by using your hand to slap the mat, which acts as a shock absorber, or dissipate the force of the fall by rolling.

You'll probably cringe as you begin observing judo students falling time and time again. Don't be turned off. Only after you've fallen on the mat a few times will you believe that falling can be accomplished without injuring yourself.

New students learn falling techniques incrementalally. Instructors usually ease them into it by having them lie on the mat with their knees bent and feet flat on the mat. With one hand gripping the belt, the other is raised close to the ear, elbow bent and palm forward. Then the arm is brought down to the side at about a thirty-degree angle to the body as the hand slaps down. Abruptly, the hand returns to the original ear position.

Next you'll slap out from a sitting position, then from a squatting position. Once you're comfortable with these positions, you'll start falling from a standing position.

After you've learned to fall, you might learn basic gripping techniques. These involve grasping the opponent's sleeve near the elbow with one hand, while the other hand grips the lapel at chest level; both sleeves or both lapels; and the sleeves with one hand while gripping the collar at the nape of the neck with the other hand.

Next you might learn how to stand when throwing someone, as well as how to prevent yourself from being thrown. To do this, you'll need to stand with your feet shoulder-width apart, knees bent slightly with the body straight and weight evenly distributed. Variations on this stance are subtle, and involve placing the right or left foot slightly forward. To keep from being thrown, you drop your body weight by bending at the knees.

When observing two judo students fighting, watch how they stand. Do they stand more or less straight while fighting, keeping their judo jackets tied down beneath their belts? Or do they crouch, with their jackets flapping about and their belts hanging down almost between their legs? If you observe the sloppier position, the school may be more concerned with winning than with technique.

Once you've tasted the basics, you're ready to throw your opponent. To accomplish this, you'll need to break your opponent's balance, move into her so she can't regain her balance, then execute the throw.

The most obvious way to throw an opponent is with your hands and feet. The foot-throwing method is perhaps the simplest and easiest to master, and one you'll probably learn first.

But hands and feet aren't the only ways to throw an opponent; hips and legs can also be used. Hip techniques involve placing your hip under your opponent's center of gravity, raising the opponent off the mat, then throwing her in a circular motion. Leg techniques usually involve sweeping or hooking the opponent's foot or leg with your own.

EXERCISES AND DRILLS

Judo training consists of three types of exercises. In one type, two students attack and defend against each other using throws, pins, chokes, and armlocks. The objective is to apply all the basic skills, including unbalancing, footwork, and timing, as well as the techniques themselves. Although this is done competitively, the objective is not to win or lose, but to improve the ability to attack and defend against an opponent.

Here, the emphasis is on correct posture, technique, footwork, and hip and body twisting. It's also on learning to train with partners of varying height and weight.

A second type of training emphasizes attack drills that stop short of performing a throw. Here, one student stands straight while the other assumes the position for the throw; however, no throw takes place. A more dynamic version of this involves both partners moving about in order to simulate a contest. The attacker continually attacks, taking her partner to the point just prior to throwing her. These exercises refine and train students in reflex and strength, increase endurance and speed, and instill confidence.

The third type of judo training embraces all the forms of throwing, grappling, and pressure-point attacks, together with cutting and thrusting with a dagger or a sword. In these prearranged routines, one student applies a technique to another student, who willingly allows the technique to be applied. The objective is to improve timing and form.

•*Karate*

As a small island situated near China and Japan, Okinawa has throughout much of its early history been the target of invaders, some of whom, while in power, confiscated and banned the use of weapons among the natives. In defense,

Okinawans developed a system of fighting using their arms and legs, as well as everyday farm tools. Thus was born karate, or "empty-handed" fighting.

The art was so effective, it was brought to Japan in the early part of the twentieth century by Gichin Funakoshi. As a result, two schools of karate developed: one in Okinawa, the other in Japan.

DIRECT AND TO THE POINT

Unlike judo, aikido, or jujitsu, karate is not a grappling art. Students learn to deliver powerful, economical kicks and strikes, and to block oncoming attacks using their arms and legs. The emphasis here is on delivering strong, perfect, accurate techniques—an element of the art that grew out of the need to stop an attacker with a single blow.

But karate emphasizes more than just simple, straightforward blows. It is a complex system of techniques that utilize just about every part of the body. Choosing what part of the hand with which to throw a simple strike, for example, becomes an exercise in and of itself. Should you strike your opponent with the knuckle of your middle finger? The tips of your forefinger and middle finger? The side of your hand? The area between your thumb and index finger? Maybe you should forget striking with your hand, and opt for the top of your wrist. And the choices go on.

Karate runs the gamut from full-force fighting to noncombative styles that focus on traditional forms and techniques. It can be aggressive and loud, characterized by hard, explosive bursts of techniques, combined with deep abdominal shouts. And it can be soft, as demonstrated through its forms, which are simply prearranged combinations of strikes, blocks, and kicks.

Karate contains three types of training. In "full-contact"

karate, well-padded students strike and kick each other with full force. A milder version of full-contact karate involves training students to control their techniques to the point where a strike or kick either stops just short of hitting the opponent or taps the opponent lightly. The third type of training involves teaching students traditional forms and techniques.

Not all schools teach all three training methods. Before joining a school, ask which methods are taught, and whether one is emphasized over the others.

STARTING WITH STANCES

As in all martial arts, balance is essential, and starts with your stance. Many karate stances distribute weight evenly, as in the traditional "sumo" stance in which the feet are spread wide and the knees are bent. Other stances, including the "cat" stance, place greater weight on the back leg, allowing the front leg ample opportunity to strike out. Then there are stances that favor the weight on the front leg to allow the student to kick straight out with the back leg.

But legs aren't just for kicking; they are just as useful for jamming or sweeping to the side an opponent's attacking leg. As with hand techniques, foot techniques utilize all parts of the leg, including the ball of the foot, side edge of the foot, heel, instep, sole, toes, and the knee.

Basic blocks are performed to defend against punches aimed at the head, midsection, or lower body. In blocking a punch, new students generally use their hand or forearm. Later, they'll extend their repertoire of blocks to incorporate both arms, then their feet and legs.

Women are usually surprised that they don't require tremendous upper body strength to throw a powerful punch. In karate, much of that strength comes from the hips. A punch begins at the hip, which shoots forward, creating a whiplash effect that forces the arm to project itself straight out. In fact, more muscular individuals often throw ineffective punches because of their bulky upper body and their tight hips.

Just as punches are generally linear, strikes are usually circular. They can be delivered with the elbow or the knee, as well as the back of the fist, bottom of the fist, side edge of the hand, and ridge part of the hand. When a strike or a punch is thrown properly, you'll hear your uniform snap, signaling that the technique had ample power and speed.

Karate kicks are almost tailor-made for women. As with punches and strikes, kicks begin in the hips. This, combined with most women's inherent flexibility makes for high, powerful kicks that are effective against even a large opponent.

New students usually begin their kicking regimen with basic versions of two kicks: snap and thrusting kicks. Snap kicks shoot out, then immediately retract, which enable the person throwing them to unleash a series in rapid succession. Thrusting kicks shoot out into the target, then lock for a second, which give the technique additional power.

In addition to these basics, new karate students learn the art of body shifting. Unlike aikido and judo, in which you stand more or less in one place, karate teaches students to move from one position to another by stepping, hopping, sliding, jumping, or turning. The goal is to become a moving target your opponent can't keep up with.

STYLES

Karate contains a variety of styles distinguishable only by minor differences. Some styles advocate low, deep traditional stances that are aesthetically pleasing, but of little practical value when fighting; other styles utilize high, mobile stances that are ideal for sparring, but aren't as dramatic.

Some styles emphasize soft moves designed to simply block an attack. Other "hard" styles utilize blocks that not only stop a strike, but injure the attacking limb as well.

Many styles, however, incorporate low and high stances, as well as hard and soft moves. One such style is Goju-ryu, an Okinawan style that translated means "hard-soft." Other popular Okinawan styles of karate are Isshin-ryu, Shorin-ryu, and Uechi-ryu. (Ryu, pronounced REE-U, means school or style.)

Goju-ryu combines hard and soft moves with circular techniques and deep abdominal breathing to create a style that is symmetrical and graceful, yet powerful and well-suited for fighting. For some students, it is the best of both worlds.

Fast, light moves typify Shorin-ryu. To keep this quick pace, the Shorin student uses high stances, and prefers hand techniques over kicks. When she does throw a kick, it's usually below the opponent's waist.

Isshin-ryu combines elements of Shorin-ryu and Goju-ryu to create a street-smart fighting art. Its notable features include unique body shifting movements, high stances, and no-nonsense techniques, including below-the-waist kicks, and snap punches and kicks.

For aggressive karate students, Uechi-ryu offers tough conditioning methods to make the body impervious to kicks and punches. In sparring, this style emphasizes strong grabbing techniques, coupled with takedowns, as well as hard kicks to the legs and midsection.

Japanese karate styles include a version of Okinawan Goju-ryu, which goes by the same name. Similar to the Okinawan version, Japanese Goju-ryu emphasizes dramatic breathing methods, and timing and speed, as well as quick, continuous punches and strikes.

Shito-ryu, Shotokan, and Wado-ryu make up the three other main styles of Japanese karate. Shito-ryu is a fairly hard style, but does incorporate soft techniques borrowed from Goju-ryu. The style also stresses the art of weaponry.

Shotokan emphasizes low, deep stances for balance, as well as direct linear attacks. Shotokan fighters are recognized by their low kicks, foot sweeps, low stances and hip power—a trademark of Japanese karate in general and Shotokan karate in particular.

Wado-ryu rejects hard physical conditioning in favor of spiritual development. Students still learn all the basics—punches, kicks, blocks, and strikes—as well as sparring and forms, but emphasis is on body shifting, and thus avoiding the full brunt of an attack.

•*Kung Fu*

Kung fu means simply skill or ability. Known in China as wushu, it is mired in religion and history. Behind it is the idea that everything in the universe consists of the same basic elements and forces, mingling and separating to produce forms of varying duration and with differing qualities.

THE NATURE OF KUNG FU

Kung fu styles tend to exhibit strenuous, energetic kicking and punching, or subtle techniques that border on being static. Though many martial arts are in some way tied to nature, none typifies nature so graphically than Chinese kung fu. Among its several hundred styles are the aptly named monkey style kung fu, white crane style, and praying mantis style. Watching students perform these styles is like watching animals come to life.

Wing chun is one of the most soft and streamlined of the martial arts. Students fight almost toe to toe, making small circular movements with their arms to catch and deflect approaching blows. Every punch, poke, strike, slap, or kick in wing chun has been designed to defend as well as attack; similarly, every block doubles as an attack.

Wing chun training contains three levels. The first consists of standing still in a narrow horse-riding stance, and practicing basic punches, parries, and blocks. The next level emphasizes defensive moves, turning the body, and delivering low kicks. The third level concentrates on open-handed finger attacks, combined with simultaneous defensive and attacking moves.

Students often work in pairs, practicing the art of "sticking hands." Here they take turns practicing techniques on each other in quick back-and-forth manner. The goal is to fine-tune reaction time, and increase upper body strength.

Training is also done on a wooden dummy consisting of a trunk, one leg, and three arms that project in different directions. It teaches the applications of trapping, controlling, and basic fighting techniques.

Jeet kune do is an offshoot of kung fu conceived in the 1960s by the late Bruce Lee, who wanted a style that incorporated a range of techniques from many styles. He believed traditional martial arts training was outdated, repetitive, and useless as a method of self-defense. As a result, jeet kune do students utilize high stances, and rarely drop their hands from their face unless it's to throw a hard, direct jab.

•Tae Kwon Do

Characterized by powerful, direct kicks, this Korean martial art translates into "kick-punch-art." Indeed, an assortment of accurate kicks and punches underscore this "hard" art, which also focuses on breaking bricks, wood, and tiles with bare hands and feet.

Tae kwon do is actually kung fu but with increased focus on acrobatic kicks that seem to almost explode off the floor. Like its kicks, tae kwon do's blocks and punches are direct and linear. Common tae kwon do kicks are the back spinning kick, round kick to the head, double jumping front kick, and jumping stamping kick.

A typical tae kwon do class includes the "basics"—linear arm blocks, punches, and kicks. As in karate, students learn forms—prearranged combinations of techniques—as well as no-contact fighting in which students face off against one another.

One of the newest forms of tae kwon do is jung suwon. As a gentler form of tae kwon do, it shies away from competition. Almost 90 percent of the moves involve kicking, making it especially appealing to women.

Unfortunately, it is taught in only one school in the United States. Its founder, Tae Yun Kim, a grandmaster with an eighth-degree black belt in tae kwon do, teaches her art in Milpitas, California. Perhaps as more women join the martial arts, jung suwon—and other, as-yet-to-be-developed, martial arts designed by women—will flourish.

•Tai Chi Chuan

Translated from Chinese, tai chi chuan means "supreme ultimate fist," and is symbolized by the familiar yin-yang symbol, which depicts the forces of light and dark intertwined. Still, most of us recognize the art as one practiced outdoors by millions of senior Chinese citizens.

What most don't realize is that this martial art is as effective a form of hard unarmed combat as it is a soft meditative exercise. Indeed, performing "Crane cools its wings," "Needle sticks at sea bottom," or any of the other memorably named moves can effectively stop an attack.

This graceful, slow-moving art is unlike any martial art. Its focus on slowing down and paying attention to the body mesmerizes some and bores others. Its admirers claim tai chi chuan improves circulation; promotes health by developing internal energy, or chi; and develops a hard, strong body.

Tai chi chuan revolves around forms, which vary in length from eighteen "postures" to more than one hundred. New students begin by learning a few postures during each lesson. Later, they'll learn prearranged routines containing these postures. When performed one after another, these postures create a balletlike dance.

•*Additional Arts:* HAPKIDO, JUJITSU, AND KENDO

Depending on where you live, you may find schools that offer additional styles of martial arts, including hapkido, jujitsu, and kendo.

Hapkido is a Korean martial art that combines aikido, judo, and karate techniques. As in aikido, hapkido utilizes wrist and joint twisting, as well as a flowing motion; as in judo, it uses throws and sweeps to gain a smooth leverage; and as in karate, the art incorporates powerful kicks and punches.

Hapkido is based on the idea of opposing forces, countering with circular movements, and penetrating an opponent's defenses. For example, if the attack is strong, it must be received gently, and likewise, if the attack is gentle, it must be countered powerfully. Reacting this way establishes a smooth, perpetual rhythm as well as constant mobility, the hallmarks of hapkido.

The Japanese art of jujitsu is based on suppleness, flexibility, and gentleness. The essence of jujitsu is the ability to move from one technique to another, or a second or even a third as needed. Techniques include kicking, striking, kneeing, throwing, choking, joint locking, and holding, as well as the use of weapons.

However, jujitsu techniques vary from school to school. One school might emphasize sword techniques, throwing techniques, and kick boxing. Another might focus on aikido combined with karate weapons. In their search for variety, jujitsu instructors have even been known to borrow ideas from ninja training and from wrestling.

Known as the "way of the sword," kendo is a traditional Japanese type of fencing. Practitioners wear samurai dress—a divided skirt worn with an apron, and a jacket worn tucked into the trousers—and use a "sword" made from strips of bamboo held together with cord and leather. Beginners are taught how to hold the sword and move in order to strike with maximum speed and efficiency.

Martial Arts and Self-Defense

A final word on choosing a style. As mentioned earlier in this chapter, in addition to the health, aesthetic, and mental benefits of taking up a martial art, many women pursue the sport under the mistaken belief that they will learn to protect themselves. If your number-one reason for signing up is to protect yourself, you should explore both martial arts and self-defense classes. Generally, most martial arts courses do not prepare students to protect themselves on the streets. Tae kwon do and karate techniques, for example, take years to learn and are too choreographed to be of much use on the street. As such, they are not effective ways for the average person to quickly master techniques for self-protection.

Self-defense classes teach women to free themselves from the grip of an attacker by using their teeth, palms, elbows, and legs to bite, strike, punch, and kick themselves free. They also teach women how to be alert to danger, carry oneself on the street, and scream effectively.

Self-defense courses generally run for several weeks. A martial arts program has no end; the more you learn, the more questions you'll have. The key is to find the art that suits you, then incorporate it into your life.

3. What to Look for in an Instructor

NOW THAT YOU HAVE a basic feel for the styles of martial arts available, it's time to move another step closer to practicing this sport. Just as it is important to find a style that suits you, it is equally important to find an instructor who suits your style.

As described in Chapter 1, the martial arts originated from the need to protect oneself. Those who didn't excel in these arts didn't survive. As the need for self-protection abated, the focus shifted to the spiritual aspects of the arts. Even so, some schools continued to focus on combative training methods. Beginning students in these schools were simply told to copy senior students. If you were lucky, your instruction might include limited verbal commands followed by a hard kick or punch intended to leave a lasting impression. In these schools, students dropped out after three months, or stayed and became lean, mean fighting machines.

Gradually, more martial arts schools began to focus on health and fitness. The move ensured schools a steady stream of students, most of whom stayed longer than three months. It also ensured schools a steady stream of revenues—a situation that spurred the proliferation of martial arts schools.

Compared to other segments of the health and fitness industry, the martial arts is fragmented. Exactly how large it is remains open to debate. *Peak Performance*, a market research newsletter for health and athletic clubs published in Bellevue, Washington, estimates that there are about 7,000 schools, including classes offered by YMCAs.

Few disagree, however, that the industry is profitable.

The martial arts industry has been estimated to produce annual revenues of $720 million to $900 million from monthly tuition fees alone. The market for equipment has been estimated at $2 billion. The franchise phenomenon has also taken hold within the martial arts. In fact, some chains have as many as 100 franchise studios, and produce revenues of $10 million and up.

Most of a martial arts school's revenue comes from monthly tuition fees. But many schools today earn income from selling equipment and uniforms, sponsoring tournaments, and charging testing fees each time a student tries to qualify for a higher belt. (In the Orient, students are usually classified as white or black belts—novice or expert. In the United States, students wear one of a range of colored belts—from white to yellow to purple to black—each of which can come with a testing fee.)

Since there is no national certifying organization for martial arts instructors, and therefore no industrywide standards, the martial arts community has little control over the quality of teaching and the awarding of belts. Though tae kwon do and judo have governing bodies because they are Olympic sports, schools are not required to join.

MARTIAL MAXIM: A WELL-TAUGHT MARTIAL ART BUILDS STRENGTH AND STAMINA IN ITS PRACTITIONERS; A POORLY COACHED MARTIAL ART CAN CAUSE SERIOUS LONG-TERM INJURIES.

To keep students, some schools have cut the time it takes to achieve a black belt. Students generally earn black belts in three to five years. But some schools today promise it in as little as one year to attract students.

As a result, the martial arts has become flooded with first-degree black belts with varying levels of ability. Within the black belt community, too, is a burgeoning number of practitioners with advance degrees. For example, whereas there should be only a handful of tenth-degree black belts—one of the highest achievable black-belt levels—there are hundreds in the United States alone.

Though the proliferation of black belts has eroded their significance, there are well-qualified eighth-, ninth-, and tenth-degree black belts in this country. Still, be wary of instructors who flaunt their black-belt ranking, and who call themselves "master" or "grand master"—titles reserved for top coaches with international reputations. You probably don't want to rule out a school solely on that basis, but keep in mind that the school may be overly concerned with marketing and reputation.

Assessing Character

Nothing defines a martial arts school more than its instructor. In fact, the instructor often *is* the school. He gives it its character—and every martial arts school has a definite character. It can be strict or unstructured, friendly or unsocial, excited or low-key, or just about any combination of characteristics. Observing just one class and meeting with the instructor can go a long way in revealing those personality traits.

One way to assess a school's character is to take a class; another is to observe one. Not all schools allow potential students to observe classes. Often they'll require them to pay for, and take one or two, trial classes. While this seems to be a growing trend among schools, with the intense competition among the various martial arts studios, it may be possible to get around this requirement. Certainly, observing is a simpler, less stressful way to assess a school and its instructor.

Flip through the yellow pages to find martial arts schools in your area. You'll probably find schools listed under "karate." Then make a list of the schools you'd like to visit. If you know someone who trains, ask them where they study and what they like and don't like about the school. Indeed, word of mouth is a strong advertising tool for any instructor. Remember the *Black Belt* survey of forty female martial artists? Twenty-five percent of them joined a martial arts school because a family member or friend was already enrolled and enjoyed the training.

Even if you're sure you've decided on a particular style, check out some others. Styles vary from school to school, from teacher to teacher. You'll be surprised how differently, say, aikido is taught at one school compared to another. In fact, it might appear to be two different styles. That's because the techniques taught in any particular school depend on the instructor's training background.

In addition, instructors often enhance their training by studying additional martial arts. Some instructors might even incorporate them into their lessons. The result is schools that don't teach pure forms but a mix of martial arts. You might be watching a karate class in progress, and notice that students are practicing moves in which one student grabs another student's wrist, then throws her to the ground—an aikido technique. Perhaps the instructor is studying aikido and incorporating it into his lessons.

MARTIAL MAXIM: MANY MARTIAL ARTS STYLES WERE CREATED BY BLACK-BELT INSTRUCTORS SEEKING THEIR OWN FAME AND FORTUNE.

Because of this melting pot of styles, it's best to visit at least five schools if you can—even if they're all karate schools.

At least you'll have other schools to fall back on if the one you choose doesn't work out.

Call a school on your list. Tell whomever answers that you're interested in the school and would like to observe a beginner class. Some schools offer beginner and advanced classes, as well as classes in which all students train, regardless of rank. On the other hand, some schools hold only the latter type of classes. I appreciated the fact that in my early training, my school offered beginner classes once a week for white and yellow belts.

When you call a school, ask with whom you're speaking. Is it an instructor or a student? You're better off speaking with the school's head instructor—the school may have just one instructor, the owner; or it may have several who work for the owner.

At this point, however, you needn't ask specific questions. Save those for when you visit the school. Stick to such general questions as how long the school has been around, the cost of membership, what time classes start, and how long they run. By asking just a few general questions, you'll learn a little about the school, and get an idea of what the instructor is like.

Choose the type of class—beginner preferably; mixed if there is no beginner class—you'd like to observe. Then set the time and day you will visit the school. That way, the instructor can, and should, be prepared to sit down with you before or after class. He—and in most cases, it will be a "he"—should also plan the class accordingly, selecting techniques and exercises that typify a beginner class.

Avoid the temptation to bring a friend. Unless your friend is interested in joining, too, she'll probably be bored and keep you from properly observing the class.

When you arrive at the school, check out its surroundings before entering. Are they safe? Well lit? I remember visiting one school, and having to drive down a long, narrow dirt driveway to a parking lot behind the school. Not only was parking tight and limited, but there were no lights. Was the instructor trying to improve students' ability to move about in the dark? Was he creating an inviting place for attackers to test their skills against those of his pupils? Was it simply a matter of a burned-out bulb? Whatever the reason, I was immediately put off, and almost didn't bother entering the school.

Once you're inside the school, take a good long look around. It should be clean, neat, and odor-free. It should also be well-lit, and the temperature should be comfortable. If it's hot outside, the air conditioning shouldn't be on full blast—cold air prevents muscles from stretching and can even tear them.

Observe the students. Do they bow before stepping on the training floor? If they do, that's a sign that the school adheres to traditional rules. Do students bow to one another? That too is a sign that traditional rules are observed.

Before class officially begins, students should be working with one another or stretching out on their own. Talk should be kept to a minimum, and should be limited to instructional advice. If you observe loud talking and fooling around, it's a sign that discipline is lacking. This is not to say that even in schools where discipline is stressed that students don't get loud. My instructor remedies this by ordering the class to do push-ups before class begins. After several of these instances, students get the message.

Notice the appearance of the students and their uniforms. You'll be coming into close contact with all of the students at some point if you join the school. Uniforms should be clean and belts should be tied neatly. Long hair should be tied back, and except for wedding bands, no one should be wearing jewelry.

Most schools I've seen have sitting areas off to the side of the training floor where potential students can observe class.

However, one school I visited allowed potential students to sit on a bench in the same room where classes were taught. Though off to the side, I felt as if the students were observing me rather than vice versa. During class, the instructor would even encourage me to attempt to duplicate a stance and throw a punch. While I appreciated the time he spent with me during his class, I would have rather remained a nonparticipating observer.

MARTIAL MAXIM: THE TRAINING FLOOR SHOULD BE MATTED OR SPRUNG, ADEQUATE FULL-LENGTH WALL MIRRORS SHOULD BE PROVIDED, AND THERE SHOULD BE NO OBSTRUCTIONS SUCH AS PILLARS, STAIRS, OR FURNITURE.

When you enter the school, don't take it upon yourself to find the instructor. Walking in anything other than bare feet in certain areas of a martial arts school is a definite no-no. Get the attention of one of the students. Tell her who you spoke with on the phone, and that you're here to observe the class. The student will either get the person with whom you spoke, or someone else who can help you, and show you from where you can observe the class. The level of courtesy extended to you is another telltale sign of the school's character.

Since you will have called, the instructor should be expecting you, and should therefore extend you the courtesy of at least stopping by to say hello. He may sit down with you and tell you a little about the class you're about to watch. Take this opportunity to observe his personality. Is it one you think you'd be comfortable with? Is he laid back or nervous? Does he speak clearly? You'll be taking a lot of instruction from him if you join the school, so you must be able to understand him. Is he in shape? If he's not, how will you learn technique if he can't perform the moves properly?

When the instructor walks on the floor, notice how students react. At this point, no one should be talking. They should be anticipating his command to line up according to rank. After they've lined up, the instructor will often give the command to bow and then sit, followed by a short meditative period during which students breathe quietly and empty their minds of the day's events.

Notice if the class started on time. That's an important sign of how well the school is run. Also, notice how students who arrive late are treated. Some instructors understand that students will be late and simply allow them to join the class—though usually behind the newest student in the back of the room so as not to disturb the rest of the class. Others might have the student do push-ups as a form of punishment. Which school would you want to belong to?

Warming-Up to a Class

Classes generally begin with warm-ups. The goal here is to raise students' heart rates, and loosen and stretch their muscles. The warm-up should take into account the training planned for the lesson. For example, a class that will involve a great deal of kicking demands a warm-up with lots of leg stretches. In many cases, the instructor will not tell the class what they'll be practicing. Therefore, the warm-up is like a radar signal that detects what's ahead.

However, just because a class will consist of kicks doesn't mean the rest of the body shouldn't be warmed up. Neck roles, push-ups, hip rotations, knee rotations, and even feet exercises are necessary to avoid injuries. Also, observe the degree of warm-ups. Are they so tough that most students can't keep up? If twenty push-ups are too much for some students, are they allowed to stop? Are they encouraged to do something else such as sit-ups? Can they finish the rest of the push-ups using their knees rather than their toes for support?

MARTIAL MAXIM: THE WARM-UP PREPARES STUDENTS TO PERFORM THE HARD, SUDDEN MOVEMENTS COMMONLY FOUND IN MARTIAL ARTS PROGRAMS.

If you're observing an evening class, most of the students will have had a full day at work or school and are justifiably tired. A good instructor uses the warm-up period to motivate. He pushes students to try harder, but doesn't fatigue them. He radiates enthusiasm—and it's contagious. He reminds them to breathe properly to keep them from tiring. At the end of the warm-up, students' energy levels are high, and they're anxious to begin class.

Observe students as they warm up. They should do the warm-up exercises in synch with one another, breathing properly and, if the instructor commands it, counting aloud. Their eyes should be focused straight ahead, and their demeanor should show concentration and determination. Rolling eyes are a sign that they're unmotivated. Laughing is a sign that they're not serious about their art. Exasperation is a sign that the warm-up is too tough, and a bored look means the warm-up isn't challenging enough.

While you're at it, notice if many of the students have injuries. Though just about every martial arts student incurs an occasional injury, numerous students with bandaged ankles and wrists and taped fingers could be a sign of a careless instructor. If a student has a slight injury, the instructor should allow the student to forgo any exercise that stresses the injured limb.

After warming up, the instructor can take any of a number of approaches. He can have the class perform drills of blocks, punches, and kicks; practice their forms; spar; or perform self-defense techniques on one another. Whatever approach is taken, you'll want to start focusing your attention on the instructor.

Center of Attention

The instructor is clearly the center of the school—his actions and words define it—which is why no two schools are alike. But just because instructors are different, doesn't mean there aren't similar traits competent ones should exhibit. Following are six traits you should observe in a good martial arts instructor.

Gives the class structure. Throwing kicks and punches for the sake of throwing them is a waste of time. A good instructor plans his class. One instruction becomes a logical extension of the previous one. He may have students do drills of punches and blocks, then have students work in pairs, one student throwing the punches she just performed, the other student blocking those punches with the blocks she performed in the drill.

Later during the class, the teacher might have students incorporate those techniques during a slow round of sparring. Then he'll have the students build up speed until they, or at least the high-ranking belts, can perform the techniques quickly and accurately. Toward the end of class, the instructor may explain the importance of understanding how to apply basic blocks and punches. The result is a well-rounded class with a definite beginning and logical conclusion.

Communicates effectively. An instructor's ability to evoke respect and loyalty from his students begins with his ability to communicate. Certainly, the instructor should speak clearly and loudly. The trick for the instructor is to do this without sounding like a drill sergeant. This is no small feat considering that it's not unusual to have twenty or more students in a class, and new students—those who require the most instruction—often find themselves in the back of the room.

The teacher's instructions should be specific. If the class cannot follow the instructions, it's probably not the students' fault. For instance, after the instructor issues a command, students should, without hesitation, implement those instructions. Do they instead look at one another, not knowing what to do?

A good instructor intersperses criticisms with positive comments. The student who continually drops her hands during sparring is told to keep her hands up to protect her face. But as she spars, the instructor should also point out areas in which she has improved. He also phrases criticisms in a positive way. Saying a kick could be higher is preferable to telling the student she kicks too low.

Finally, the effective communicator doesn't do all the talking. Teaching is a give-and-take exercise. While the teacher will, and should, do most of the talking, students should feel free to ask questions. The teacher in turn should take each question seriously. That involves taking the time to ensure that everyone heard the question, then explaining and perhaps demonstrating the issue until everyone understands.

Maintains control of the class. Maintaining control of a class doesn't mean ruling with an iron fist. However, it does mean that the instructor's comments and commands are reacted to immediately. If students are sparring and the instructor calls the class's attention to a pair of students who are sparring together particularly well, all students should immediately stop what they're doing and direct their attention to the instructor.

Control is also maintained by keeping the full attention of the class. To that end, the instructor never stays in one place too long. He constantly moves about, demonstrating a technique from different angles so all students see it. To keep students on their toes, he may randomly select one to help him demonstrate a technique.

By maintaining control, the instructor also limits the amount and types of injuries. For example, when instructing pairs of students to implement a throw, an astute instructor foresees what could go wrong, and plans for it. He'll make sure mats are plentiful and positioned correctly. New students won't be paired with other beginners, and the technique will be demonstrated enough times so everyone understands its basic premise.

Finally, the instructor should be able to handle a crisis situation calmly and professionally. If a student gets injured or starts to feel sick, the instructor should see to the injured student's needs while keeping the rest of the class calm.

Focuses on students' individual needs. A competent instructor understands that students are individuals. Some have a great deal of strength, others more flexibility. Some have quick reaction times, others are slow to react. The instructor recognizes each student's strong and weak points, and trains accordingly.

Some students take a martial art to spar and compete; others to focus on traditional forms. Instructors can and should be able to contour a class to provide training that satisfies both types of students. During sparring exercises, the instructor might push competition-oriented students harder, pairing them up with the best fighters. During forms training, the instructor might push traditional-oriented students harder, stressing deeper stances and fine-tuning timing.

Surely, creating the feeling that one-on-one training is taking place within a class environment is difficult. But a good instructor can do it. He'll mix general instructions with specific comments and criticisms directed at individual students. When this is done effectively, students will finish class feeling as though they are better at their art than before class began.

Treats students equally. You probably won't find schools whose student populations are predominately female. Don't be discouraged. Rather than focusing on the number of female students in the class, direct your attention to how the ones who are present are treated. You shouldn't notice any difference.

Women don't have the same physical abilities as men, and vice versa. Female students may be more flexible, and male students stronger (though, of course, there are exceptions). Nevertheless, female and male students are expected to try to perform all the techniques, even the ones with which they have difficulty. Every student—male and female—has his or her own limitations, and the instructor should know those limits.

Consequently, it's not a question of male or female, but of individual students, each of whom excels in some aspects of the art and lags behind in others. For example, I do well in forms and in technique; sparring and applying techniques are another matter. For some women, the opposite is true.

Just as instructors walk a fine line between treating female and male students equally, they also have to contend with treating high-ranking students the same as new students. Instructors will often call on high-ranking students to correct new students. While this type of instruction is common, it shouldn't replace instruction that comes directly from the teacher, and it certainly shouldn't be done so the instructor can dwell on certain students.

Teaches more than technique. A good instructor tells students not only how to perform a technique, but why they are performing it. For example, to the uninformed student, forms are just a bunch of techniques strung together. To the well-learned student, each move in a form represents a reaction to a grab, punch, kick, or strike.

The instructor also incorporates the history and terminology of his style into the curriculum. Not all instructors teach the history of their martial art style, and it's up to you if that's an aspect of your training you want to pursue. If it is, you'll want to look for a teacher who sprinkles his instruction with references to the style's founder and the events that led the founder to develop the style.

Traditional instructors generally expect their students to know who developed a style, why it was developed, and where it was developed. In addition to history, terminology in traditional schools is often stressed. Karate students, for example, would learn the Japanese terms for every technique and form. They would also learn to count in Japanese, and greet one another with the traditional Japanese greeting, "Oss," rather than its English equivalent, "How are you?"

Staying After Class

Just as classes begin with warm-ups, they end with cool-downs. During the cool-down period, the instructor puts students through a series of slow exercises and gentle stretches designed to return the heart rate to normal. Afterward, as students leave the floor, notice how they appear. If the workout was challenging and productive, you'll notice that the students appear energized. The combination of having endured a tough workout and improved technique is powerful, and it doesn't happen unless the teacher made it happen.

As students leave the training floor, don't approach them to ask about the school. Students don't want to be put in the awkward position of having to talk about the school to a stranger in front of their peers.

Just stay put. The instructor will more than likely approach you to see if you have questions. Though you're bound to have your own, here are a few to get you started.

How are the classes broken up, and what's the average number of students per class?

It's reassuring to know you can attend a beginner class. It relieves the pressure of having to perform with high-ranking belts, and it allows new students to build self-confidence. But don't be discouraged if only mixed classes are offered. In this case, when you observe a class, pay particular attention to the beginners, and note if they appear at ease amid the rest of the students.

The number of students per class can vary. If there is one instructor per class, it probably shouldn't contain more than twenty students. However, some classes contain more than one instructor, and in that case, there could be as many as thirty students.

Do you teach the history and terminology of your style of martial art?

If you couldn't tell from the class you observed, and you're interested in this aspect, by all means ask.

How many women are in your school?

Certainly, there is no magic number that tells you this is a great school for women. I attended a school in which I was the only female—a situation that made little difference in my training. However, if the instructor responds to the question with something like, "Women join, but they all drop out after a month," you may want to rethink the school.

A better question might be, Has your school produced any female black belts? This will tell you whether the instructor's female students liked the school enough to stay for several years. You might even want to follow up this question with, Do they still train here? Since many students quit after attaining their black belt, it's a good school that can keep them after this period of their training.

If I don't like sparring, do I have to do it?

Chances are you'll have to spar whether you want to or not. But a good instructor will allay any fears or reservations you might have by telling you that new students aren't thrown into sparring. Initially, new students watch sparring matches in class. Then they'll be eased into it by working slowly with a high-ranking student. Not until you've been promoted at least once will you be sparring with any force. By then, you'll probably have lost much of your reservations about sparring.

Does your school participate in competitions?

Usually a glance in the school's front window or trophy case will answer this question, but ask it anyway. Some schools strongly encourage their students to compete in tournaments. Others don't push students at all, but will help students train if they want to compete.

How does your school compare to others in the area?

The instructor should be able to tell you if there are other schools in the area that teach the same style he does. There might be ten karate schools in your area, and two that teach a style, say Goju-ryu, that you are interested in studying. If that's the case, he should tell you.

He should also be able to tell you how his school differs from others in the area, and what makes his school better. It's no secret that martial arts instructors spy on one another's schools. If the instructor can't go to a school posing as a potential student, he is likely to send one of his own students. The practice is widespread, and there's nothing wrong with it. If anything, it benefits students because instructors are always trying to improve their schools.

Can I take a trial class?

Don't ask this question unless you liked enough of what

you just saw to take a class. And certainly don't ask this question first. It will make you appear as though you are more interested in getting a free class than studying a martial art. If you are interested in the style, school, and the instructor, then by all means ask if you can take a trial class. In many cases, if the instructor sees that you're enthusiastic and serious about joining, he'll make the offer first.

If I decide to take a few classes, do I have to buy a uniform, or can I wear sweats?

You don't want to buy a uniform if you decide to train in a different school from the one you observed. Just as there are different styles of martial arts, there are different styles of uniforms. First make sure you want to train at a particular school. Then ask the instructor what style of uniform you should purchase.

How many times a week can I attend class?

Some instructors allow students to attend any class they want as many times per week as they want. Others limit students to a set number of classes. Since the average class is from one to two hours long, the instructor will probably recommend you train three times a week.

Once a week won't do much except leave you sore and slow your level of improvement to a crawl. Twice a week will keep you conditioned, but you won't improve fast enough to maintain a high level of interest. Three times a week will keep you in great shape, do wonders for your technique, and allow your body ample time to rest in between.

What costs can I expect to incur if I join your school?

Schools usually charge a monthly fee, which can start at $55 and go up. On the other hand, some schools charge a flat fee for an entire training program—from white to black belt. Payments are generally made in installments. My school charges a monthly fee of $65, with no testing fees. For years, black belt students paid only $35 per month, but were occasionally required to assist the instructor with new students during class. But in a sign of the tough economic times schools have gone through, black belts in my school now pay full price.

As with any purchasing decision, be wary of long-term contracts and hefty up-front fees. What incentive is there for an instructor to keep you happy if he has all your money up-front?

In addition, schools will eventually require you to purchase a uniform, which can cost as much as $75, as well as equipment, which can easily run up to $100 for foot and shin pads, forearm guards, gloves, and head gear. Many schools also charge fees of about $25 every time a student is tested for a promotion. For schools that sponsor tournaments, participating students generally pay $25 to compete.

Negotiate

Before you leave, tell the instructor what aspects of the class you liked most. He might say that if you joined, he would incorporate more of that into your training. Take him up on the offer. Too often, instructors make such an offer only after a student decides to stop training.

Certainly, martial arts instructors are faced with a dilemma: Maintaining the delicate balance between training students hard enough to keep them interested, but not too hard to discourage them. This combined with the fact that most classes include students at different levels of expertise makes the balance even more difficult to achieve.

But it can be done, and it all comes down to the instructor. Putting a little effort into choosing one will make your martial arts training rewarding and productive.

HOW ONE WOMAN'S PASSION TURNED INTO THE KARATE SCHOOL FOR WOMEN

Anyone who has ever studied a martial art has at one time or another questioned—whether silently to themselves or openly with their fellow students—the teaching methods of their instructor. And because women stand a good chance of being in a male-dominated class taught by a male teacher, they might even be among the more inclined to disagree with how class is conducted. "If only I were an instructor, I would teach class this way ..." goes the thinking.

Well, one woman did more than just think about it. Since 1976, Roberta Schine has operated the Karate School for Women in New York City where she teaches tae kwon do. Today, she holds a second-degree black belt in tae kwon do and is a certified Kripalu yoga instructor. She teaches yoga at her school and to people with cancer at SHARE, a self-help organization for women with breast and ovarian cancer, and at Memorial Sloan-Kettering Cancer Center in New York. [SHARE is located at 19 West 44th Street, Suite 415, New York, NY 10036; 212-719-0364.]

Here, Schine discusses how and why she started her school.

Why a karate school for women?

I had been studying karate in New York in a traditional karate school that had about seventy men and four women. Most of the women were somebody's wife or girlfriend, or they were very athletic. I was none of the above.

I thought, "If I were doing this, I would teach it this way." For example, when it was time to fight, the teacher would say, "Bow, begin." I didn't have the experience to know what to do. In my family, we weren't encouraged to be physical.

When I first started sparring, all I could think about was not getting hurt. It was the same with the other women. After a while, I thought, "If I were teaching this class, I would have one woman hit slowly, then the other would block slowly." In that way, they could see what was happening, and they wouldn't be scared.

How did the school come about?

I met a few women in town who studied karate. We all just seemed to meet by accident. One woman I know who was studying a martial art noticed another woman on the subway whose [martial arts] belt was sticking out of her bag, so she started talking to her. They decided to start meeting, and I was invited to the original meeting in 1973.

These meetings went on for four years, and included anywhere from eight to fifteen women. We called ourselves the Women's Martial Arts Union. Eventually, we found out that similar groups were forming all over the country, and we began meeting and training together. In 1981, we became the National Women's Martial Arts Federation, and today there are about 1,000 members.

[The National Women's Martial Arts Federation can be reached at P.O. Box 820, Kings Park, NY 11754, Attention Dara Masi; 516-261-4229.]

What went on at these meetings?

At first we talked a lot. We complained about our schools, and we supported one another because many of the women were on the brink of quitting. We were all attending schools and fighting and feeling frustrated. We were being ignored, laughed at, humiliated when we made mistakes, neglected, or hit a little too hard when we fought. In some schools, the men wouldn't even fight with the women.

So we helped one another figure out strategies for surviving in our schools. We fantasized about what it would be like if we had all-women classes. For example, if we were teaching, we would offer women advice on how to do knuckle push-ups without hurting themselves. We would also come up with ideas to help women lose their fear of fighting. We would have hitting exercises—one woman would say, "On a scale of one to ten, you can hit me a two." This promoted a feeling of being in control. If someone cried, we talked about how she felt. It was a woman's way of learning to feel strong.

How did the meetings progress from there?

During the second year, we started working out with each other—in someone's apartment or at community centers where some of the women had jobs. Later we practiced in the park, but crowds would form so we stopped.

During our third year, three women started their own schools, and they attracted students very easily. Around that time, I got a call from someone at Richmond College (in Staten Island, New York), saying they'd like to offer a special karate class for women during Christmas break. I said I knew some men who could teach it, and they said, "No, we want you to teach it." I said, "Oh my God." My support group said great.

When I asked my teacher if I could teach in Richmond College's Women's Studies Department, he responded as if it were unthinkable. He muttered something about women, and then he actually burst out laughing. And he said, "Absolutely not." So I changed my name to "Florence Flowerpot" and I've been teaching karate to women ever since. Eventually he did find out I was teaching women-only classes, but by that time I was bringing him students to be tested, and hence money, so that matter was dropped.

I think his objection to my teaching was partly because I was a woman and partly because I was only a purple belt (an intermediate level) at the time. He didn't understand that women were desperate to learn the martial arts from other women. The level of skill of the teacher was not so important in those days. As long as I knew more than the students, I had something to teach.

What was that experience like?

At the first class, some women came in nylon stockings, and one even wore a hat with a veil. I could not get women to take off their panty hose. The second day, one student—the dean's wife—fell and broke her arm. Still, they hired me right away next semester, but budget cuts ended that a year or so later.

After that I got a job teaching karate at New York University. On the first day I came to teach class, I was given a list of twelve or thirteen students who had signed up. But when I got there, there were fifty students—the Richmond College students had snuck in!

Eventually women wanted to train more than once a week, and we began renting space wherever we could: in a dance studio, in back of a primal therapy loft where people were screaming in the next room, in a church basement. Then, in 1976, I had the opportunity to have my own loft in Greenwich Village, and we have been there ever since.

Sparring seems to be a particularly contentious area for women. How do you teach it in your school?

White belts don't spar in my school. They concentrate on getting stronger and faster, and they learn basic concepts. After about six months, they earn their yellow belts and then start sparring. But we start with basic exercises. I teach students a punch and a block, and we do it in slow motion. This helps them get beyond their fears. I might have them improve their rhythm by having them move to a drumbeat. I'll also use red dots positioned on someone's gi and say, "Punch ten times to the top dot, ten to the middle, then ten to the lower one."

Do any of your students spar competitively?

Some of my students compete. And when they do they do well, because so much of it comes from the inner self.

Tae kwon do is one of the harder styles of martial arts, especially compared to softer styles such as tai chi chuan and aikido. Why do you think women are attracted to tae kwon do?

Tae kwon do is simply a harder style of karate. I think that's why women like it. It's something they've traditionally been barred from experiencing. They want to know what it's really like to yell and stomp.

I think women have more endurance than men, and research is bearing this out. We do seem to have more longevity. I don't know *why, but in my experience, men often get good very quickly and then you don't see them again. They stop coming. Men tend to quit when they get injured; women modify what they are doing.*

Do your students interact with male martial artists?

Yes. Shortly after I received my second-degree belt, I began training with Michael Bradshaw, a wonderful martial artist, at his school in Red Bank, New Jersey. He would sometimes bring men to my school, or I would bring my students to his school.

What else do you do at your school?

I teach both yoga and karate. They go well together because both are about energy, but at different ends of the spectrum. And they're both about integration of mind and body. For karate students, yoga helps increase flexibility and avoid injuries.

For two years, I have been teaching yoga to women with breast cancer. Being a breast cancer survivor myself, I feel very connected with this work. I teach women to use yoga and meditation as an important adjunct to their treatment. I recently watched Bill Moyers's Healing *and the* Mind, *which featured one segment about a doctor who studied eighty-six women with breast cancer. Half of them had standard treatment; the other half added yoga and group therapy. The results were astounding. They found a huge difference in the second group's quality and length of life. Yoga has been practiced for 4,500 years, so this has been well understood in the East for thousands of years.*

Do you see a trend of more schools for women?

There are already lots of schools for women. Some mixed schools have classes reserved just for women. Many are changing because more male instructors are learning how to properly teach women students. But for many women there will always be a special approach that exists in an all-women's school, which makes learning karate a profound and exhilarating experience.

4. What Students Are Expected to Learn

JUST AS STUDENTS ENTER the martial arts with expectations of a school and an instructor, martial arts instructors have expectations of their students.

A martial arts school is, in most cases, a business. (Few martial artists can afford to run a school simply for enjoyment and fulfillment.) As such, the owner, who is oftentimes the head instructor, wants his school to look professional—right down to its students. To that extent, he wants students who are serious about training, have a desire to learn and a positive attitude, and are in fairly good physical shape. After all, as a student, you are an example of what the school can do for prospective students.

Once you start training, the instructor's expectations will only increase. Physically, students are expected to try to keep up with what can at times be demanding workouts. Warm-ups alone can be draining. On top of that, you'll be expected to learn forms and self-defense techniques, and perhaps sparring and classical weapons training.

Mentally, students are expected to take their training seriously and adhere to the rules of the school and the instructor. Though rules differ from school to school, there are basic ones that every school follows. (Chapter 6 details basic rules pertaining to female students.) Suffice it to say, however, that learning to respect the rules is as important as learning to do a flying kick or to slap out from a roll.

Students are also expected to use their minds to make themselves better martial artists. The abilities to clear one's mind before class, to plan a move, to perform before a crowd, to understand how and why a technique is performed, and to push oneself to do more are mental strengths the martial arts seeks to develop among its practitioners.

Effort Counts

Half the battle of studying a martial art is pushing yourself to be in the best shape you can—and if you don't push yourself, your instructor will. That's not to say you'll be ridiculed if you can't do twenty push-ups in a row, or if you can't fall gracefully into a split. But you are expected to try. Attitude counts almost as much as physical ability. Put effort into your workout, and you'll build strength, increase stamina and speed, and improve flexibility beyond your own expectations.

Indeed, strength, stamina, speed, and flexibility are the building blocks of the martial arts. Understanding the role they play in training will help you understand the physical characteristics that make up just about every style of martial art.

In the martial arts, strength is developed through warm-up exercises performed before class, as well as through drills practiced during class. A common misunderstanding among nonmartial artists is that bulk equals strength. It doesn't in this sport. Look at any martial arts veteran; you won't see strength, although you know it's there. You could feel it if she were to punch you, grab your wrist, or sweep you with her foot. You can see it as she spars; the fast, hard techniques she wields, as well as the control she exercises as she throws a punch that stops just short of hitting her opponent. You can also hear strength. Listen as students perform punching drills. When done correctly, their uniforms will "snap" every time they unleash a punch.

Bulk is not only unnecessary in the martial arts, but can actually be a drawback because it tends to decrease flexibility. Still, some students continue to pump up at the gym, then come to class expecting to be the star pupil. But for every inch they gain in their physique, they lose in terms of flexibility— a trait as important in the martial arts as strength. When you observe a class, look for a muscular type and watch how he performs. If he's sparring, for example, his kicks are probably low, and he doesn't use his hips to help propel his punches. He probably stands in one place and throws a punch or two whenever the opponent comes in. He's like a punching bag with arms. This is not the martial arts.

Female students shouldn't be impressed or intimidated by their muscular martial arts counterparts. When you're paired with a muscle-bound student, use speed and timing to avoid hits from him. As he withdraws a technique, come in and throw your own, then get out. Keep in mind, however, that muscular students may not have the control to stop a technique just short of hitting a target. Taking a hit from one of these students will almost surely result in an injury. You're not expected to take this. If you're paired with a student whom you think can't control his techniques, keep your distance and don't take chances. Wait until you're paired with someone you trust.

Certainly, you're not expected to risk injuring yourself in the name of excelling in the martial arts. However, it's easy to get so caught up in your training that you take chances you wouldn't normally take. It's also common to allow your training to become all-consuming. There is a strong element of competition within most schools. Students who start training to learn something new and stay in shape soon become caught up in the pressure to not only keep up but excel.

But while no student is expected to be the best and the brightest, many nevertheless go to great lengths to achieve that status. To that extent, they'll supplement their training by joining a gym or health club, or running or cycling. Admittedly, when I started my martial arts training, as a former health club attendee, I was struck by the absence of weights and Nautilus equipment in my karate school. The training floor was barren, except for some punching bags and pads. Instead of interacting with machines and objects, students, for the most part, work with each other. What soon became apparent is that you don't need steel and iron to build strength; the resistance generated between two human beings is as effective in building muscle as pressing weights.

When done properly, working out with weights can improve strength, while not limiting flexibility. Some schools even make weights available to students. Years ago, I invested in a set of six-pound free weights, which I use while watching television. The reps I did conditioned me so that I could better keep up with push-ups and other in-class warm-up exercises.

I also took up running. Although I never ran more than three miles a week, it was enough to help me develop stamina. Unfortunately, my knees couldn't take the stress of both running and martial arts training. As a result, I limited my running to when I needed its benefits the most, which was usually several weeks before I would be tested for a promotion.

Schools that don't make weights available to students are likely to incorporate traditional training equipment into their curriculums. Chapter 7 provides an overview of these simple but effective training devices, including medicine balls, punching bags, and impact pads.

No matter how many students in your class supplement their training, don't feel pressured to do the same. Certainly, you'll run into students totally immersed in their martial arts training—taking class four times a week, training at a gym twice weekly, assisting the instructor with children's classes, and competing in tournaments. Then there will be students who attend class two or three times a week, improving at slow increments, but content with their progress.

The tendency is to get caught up in a sort of training frenzy, competing to be the strongest and fastest, and to have the most endurance. Don't let it get the best of you. Decide before you start training what role you want the martial arts to play in your life. Most of the women—from single careerists to full-time homemakers—I've trained with took up a martial art to enhance their lives, not complicate them. Neither competition nor a drive to be the star pupil attracted them to the martial arts. They attended class two or three times a week, and rarely trained outside class. Those who didn't sway from those principles were more likely to stick with their training and enjoy it.

When you consider the rigorous training a martial arts school provides, there's almost no reason to seek additional training. The basic, no-frills exercises most instructors depend on are effective. Push-ups for the upper body, sit-ups or crunches for the abdomen, and squats for the legs do wonders for strengthening and sculpting the body.

Sound boring? It might if instructors didn't add their own variations to these exercises. My instructor "enhances" push-ups by having students perform them on their fingertips—something I never mastered. Variations for sit-ups done with knees bent and feet flat on the floor include twisting so each elbow touches the opposite knee, or simply holding your torso in midair, two or three inches from the floor, for a minute or two. And because my style of martial arts incorporates kicks, the instructor has students kick as they rise from warm-up squats.

Again, remember effort. I rarely keep up when it comes to push-ups, but I try. Sometimes I lie exhausted and weak on my stomach with my forehead on the floor as others around me push up and down, up and down, and I wonder how I ever got myself in such a predicament. One exercise I never managed to perform well even once involves sitting up on the floor with both legs sticking straight out and palms flat on the floor. The idea is to raise and hold yourself off the floor using only your hands for support. But while I can't do it (I still suspect it's done with mirrors), I can honestly say I've tried.

Warm-ups are such an integral part of the martial arts that some schools become famous for them. My school's specialty includes having students drag themselves across the floor using only their hands. Lying on your stomach, you reach up with both hands, slap the floor, then pull yourself forward—using your feet is not allowed. Not only did this build the upper body, but it cleaned the floor as well!

> **MARTIAL MAXIM: THE PURPOSE OF MOST WARM-UP EXERCISES IS TO ENABLE THE BODY TO MOVE FREELY WITHIN ITS LIMITS; THE REST OF YOUR TRAINING IS INTENDED TO PUSH YOU BEYOND YOUR BODY'S LIMITS.**

While individual training is probably the most common form of martial arts training, one-on-one training is doubly effective because in addition to building strength, it familiarizes students with how to work with one another—something you'll certainly be expected to do. Again, basic exercises, some of which you may have done in gym class as a grade-school student, will once again whip you into shape. Among them: wheelbarrows, sit-ups during which one person holds your feet, and leg lifts during which one partner pushes the legs down as you bring them up. In addition, you might perform resistance training with a partner in which you both push against each other's force. While performing these exercises with a partner is physically challenging, the challenge that lies in learning to work with a partner can be just as great.

I can't think of any sport in which male and female students work as closely together as in the martial arts. While you might expect a high degree of unease among males and females to be limited to teen classes, adult classes have their share of male students who are uncomfortable working with women, and vice versa. I've seen perfectly normal, intelligent people become flustered and jittery when paired with someone of the opposite sex. I've also seen pairs of students become so aggressive during warm-ups that in their zeal to outdo each other, the workout actually becomes dangerous.

Hypothesizing about why these problems arise isn't constructive. What's important to remember is that you will be expected to work with just about every student in your class. It's not your instructor's way of acquainting students with one another; it's done for practical reasons, such as conditioning yourself to perform techniques on partners of different sizes and strengths. Keep this in mind if your instructor should ever pair you up with a six-foot, 200-pound-plus partner.

For every partner I've worked with who was easygoing and responsible, there was one who wasn't. If you encounter someone who seems more intent on competing with you than working with you, speak up. A simple "Let's take this a little slower" is usually enough to get the point across. The biggest mistake you can make is to not say anything, which is what I used to do. I often hesitated to speak up unless I was experiencing pain—and even then I'd keep quiet, thinking that it would be over soon so I might as well just endure it. Don't make the same mistake I did.

You may find yourself working with someone who isn't a threat physically, but seems uptight about working with you. In this case, try diverting your attention from whom you're working with, concentrating instead on the task at hand. By showing your partner that you are more concerned with what you're doing as opposed to who you are doing it with, the other person usually relaxes. Acquiring a knack for putting your partner at ease and making him forget he's working with a woman is a talent you'll carry over into other areas of your life.

Stamina and Speed

In addition to strength, the martial arts requires students to develop stamina and speed. Stamina gives you the staying power to perform during a drawn-out sparring match, perform roll after roll, and throw a hundred or more techniques in a row. Speed allows you to evade an on-coming opponent, block a punch or a kick, and build enough power to execute a long stunning flying kick.

Stamina and speed are great substitutes for power. What women lack in strength, they can make up for in stamina and speed. I've seen petite women dance circles around their male opponents, and get in the last punch or kick as their exhausted partner stood too tired to block it.

Common drills for building stamina include running in place while bringing the knees up as high as possible, running back and forth across the floor while throwing punches and kicks, and performing sets of block-punch-kick combinations. During these drills, instructors, in their zeal to get students to attain their best, often count faster than students can perform the moves. This is a common practice among instructors designed to push students to their maximum speed. Once in a while you'll be able to keep up; many times you won't. Don't get frustrated. Just look around you. Chances are you're doing better than a lot of the other students, including high-ranking ones.

Speed is also about timing. Developing reaction speed allows you to conserve energy and deliver fast comebacks.

Ducking an on-coming technique or jumping out of its way allows you to set yourself up to deliver a follow-up technique. Had you blocked the on-coming technique, it would have taken you more time to set yourself up to throw a follow-up technique.

In addition to strength, stamina, and speed, you'll be expected to increase your flexibility. But unlike stamina and speed drills, flexibility exercises are performed slowly. Long, deliberate stretches prevent muscles and ligaments from tearing, and train your body to execute aesthetically pleasing forms and techniques.

> MARTIAL MAXIM: NEW STUDENTS ARE GENERALLY LEAST FLEXIBLE IN THEIR HIPS, WHICH IS WHERE FLEXIBILITY IS MOST NEEDED IN ORDER TO EXECUTE HIGH KICKS, STRONG PUNCHES, AND FLAWLESS THROWS. WOMEN, HOWEVER, TEND TO BE MORE FLEXIBLE THAN MEN AS A RESULT OF THEIR SMALLER MUSCLES.

Leg stretches are one of the most common forms of exercises to improve flexibility. But as stated earlier, you don't have to be capable of performing Russian splits to excel in the martial arts. I've never done a perfect split, and most students I've trained with can't do them either. While you're expected to work on improving your ability to master a split, don't let your instructor or anyone force you to do something your body resists.

I recall when my instructor invited a well-known martial artist to our school—a common practice designed to give students a chance to meet with a martial arts celebrity, and give the celebrity exposure and pocket money. This particular martial artist is well-known for his high kicks and ability to fall quickly into splits. During class, he asked students to attempt a Russian split. He walked around the class observing us.

Then he stopped behind a student who happened to be facing me. The celebrity martial artist placed his hands on the student's shoulders and with a force that made me grimace, pushed down until the student was in a Russian split. I never saw sweat form as quickly as it did on this student's brow—it actually popped out in big fat beads. While the student wasn't injured, I seriously doubt most instructors would approve of these methods.

The Basics of Basics

Basics are the foundation of the martial arts. As such, all students, from the newest ones to black belts, are expected to study them. The theory behind this requirement is that no one can master punches, strikes, kicks, blocks, and rolls. But through continuous practice, students can come close. Here, approaching perfection is the goal—something that's done through repetition.

This theory—never being able to achieve perfection—is at the root of the martial arts. Instructors who adhere to it generally produce students who have perseverance and are patient and perhaps even humble. But these traits don't come easily. There will be times when you'll silently curse your instructor for making you practice the same technique over and over again. You'll think he has gone mad, or you're going to if you throw another kick or punch or whatever technique you are being drilled on. There were times during these drills when I despised my instructor for making me do the same combination of moves over and over again, and at top speed. But as quickly as thoughts of quitting or screaming out during class come, they go away.

MARTIAL MAXIM: STUDENTS ARE REQUIRED TO REMAIN EXPRESSIONLESS AS THEY PERFORM TECHNIQUES. THAT MEANS NO WANDERING EYES, NO LOOKS OF EXASPERATION, AND NO LAZY TONGUES STICKING OUT.

New students often report feeling clumsy compared to other students—and that's because they are. Unless you're a dancer or tightrope walker, you probably never had to do anything on one leg, or do something with your legs and something totally different with your arms. Don't get frustrated. Throwing a kick at an imaginary opponent behind you, as well as developing eye and hand coordination, doesn't come easy. But it's the first step in learning basic moves.

Contrary to what the name implies, basic moves are anything but basic. Throwing a punch is not as simple as squeezing your hand, then thrusting it forward. It involves knowing how to make a fist, where to position your elbow and shoulder, how to use your hip to strengthen the impact of the punch, when to inhale and exhale, how to place the stance, and what to do with the arm that's not punching. Add them up, and you've got a lot to think about.

Now consider that basics are comprised of not only punches, but stances, strikes, kicks, and blocks. Consider further that for each basic there are numerous variations. For example, there are straight punches, rising punches, hook punches, parallel punches, double and triple punches, reverse punches, circular punches, vertical punches, lunge punches, and more. Within any style, there could be hundreds, if not thousands, of different variations on the basics.

New students who persevere eventually get the knack of performing basics. Then it's on to combining them—performing a block and a punch consecutively, for example. Later, you'll perform three or more basics in a row.

But this process doesn't happen quickly. It could be six

months before you're ready to perform combinations of techniques. If a new student is taught a technique too early, it more often than not results in frustration. For example, learning to throw a roundhouse kick is senseless if the student hasn't developed an understanding of, and knack for, using the flexibility in her hips, or adjusting her feet so her stance is strong. What's more, basics are developed in increments. A new student being taught roundhouse kicks won't be expected to aim for her opponent's head. Rather, she'll be taught to kick low, say to the knee, then she'll work her way up to the midsection, and later the head.

Initially, you'll be throwing punches and kicks at an invisible opponent. Later, you'll be required to practice techniques with a partner. As with warm-up exercises requiring a partner, new students are expected to handle this part of their training seriously and maturely.

Practicing self-defense techniques with a partner will give you your first taste of the importance of developing a rapport with your partner. At first, you'll be teamed up with high-ranking belts (the thinking is that experienced brown and black belts will be more careful than low-ranking students). And it's true that high-ranking belts are more careful—sometimes to the point where they get hurt, not the new student.

During one class, I was asked to work with a new student—a tall, young, fairly strong male. We were working on mats, practicing some fairly complex moves that built up to a throw. I talked the new student through the move slowly to the point where he would throw me. Noticing that I wouldn't hit the mat if he continued with the throw, I told him to go no further. He continued with the technique anyway, and I ended up diving into the floor. The result? Ten stitches on my eyebrow.

Was the accident the new student's fault. No. Was it mine? Probably. If I had tucked in my head and just gone with the flow, I would have been fine. Instead, I panicked and suffered the consequences. On the other hand, maybe the technique was too advanced for this student.

Students should not feel pressured to perform a technique. If it feels too advanced, chances are it is. Keep in mind that the instructor is supervising every other student in the class, and is prone to misjudge the abilities of some of them. Tell the instructor of your apprehension. Even if he tells you to try the technique, he'll at least keep a closer eye on you.

Naturally, the chances of injury increase as you learn more complex self-defense techniques. You'll find your repertoire of techniques will grow from simple punches, blocks, and grabs to fancy foot and hand combinations and spinning jump kicks and fast, hard sweeps. This constant grabbing, pushing, and throwing takes some getting used to. People simply aren't used to, or accepting of, people who grab, pull, or push them.

During technique training you'll be grabbed by the sleeve, collar, belt, hair; subjected to having sensitive pressure points poked; grappled with until you fall to the floor; and have joints twisted and turned until you tap your partner, indicating you can no longer bear the pain and she should loosen her hold. It takes a lot of getting used to, especially when you're working with a partner who is stronger and rougher than you care for.

When students work together properly, it doesn't matter if one is half the size of the other. Self-defense techniques are done under the supervision of your instructor, who should set firm rules for these situations. He's not interested in having students injure one another because it affects his school's reputation.

As you continue your technique training, you'll discover how to fall without batting an eye, how to move smoothly in the direction of a technique, and how to signal your partner that the technique was effectively applied, and it's now time to loosen the grip or let go. The latter is done with a simple slap. Say, for example, two students are practicing wrist grabs on one another. One student grabs the wrist of her partner, who reflectively brings her hand up to her face, in effect loosening the grab, peels her opponent's fingers off her wrist, then proceeds to slowly twist the wrist of her opponent, who slaps her side or her opponent when she can no longer take the pain. Certainly, you're not required to hold your slap until you're dizzy with pain. On the other hand, you shouldn't slap before you feel anything.

As your training progresses, you'll be required to work with all students in your class—not just the high-ranking ones. The tendency among many students is to work with those students with whom they feel most comfortable. As a result, women team up with women, men with men, tall students with their tall counterparts, and so on. I've actually stood in a class of all male students as they scattered to find male partners, going out of their way to avoid having to work with me. In addition to summoning up memories of being the last team player picked in gym class, it drove home the fact that adults can be as childlike as children.

It just goes to show that people are naturally inclined to avoid situations that may make them uncomfortable. A good instructor realizes this, and will, after letting students work with their chosen partners, stop the class and have students choose new partners. Eventually, students have no choice but to work with someone of the opposite sex, or someone who is stronger or weaker, taller or shorter, or more or less aggressive than themselves.

While the tendency is to get caught up with who your partner is, it's more productive to consider what your doing. Even a relatively simple technique requires thinking about several things at once: where to move your feet, what direction to move in, which hand to grab, how to move your hips, when to add speed, when to slow down, and other numerous thoughts. On top of performing the technique accurately, you have to consider your partner, and ensure his or her safety.

When you first begin to work with a partner, chances are

he or she won't put up much, if any, resistance. You may even begin to think that this martial arts stuff is pretty easy, and that you're just naturally inclined to it. Then as you progress, you'll find that senior students don't cooperate as much, and that every time you get a little better so do they.

> **MARTIAL MAXIM: THE MARTIAL ARTS IS A LESSON IN SELF-DISCOVERY SIMPLY BECAUSE YOU'RE NOT ALLOWED TO HIDE BEHIND NERVOUS GIGGLING OR BOW OUT IF YOU'RE NOT INTERESTED IN ATTEMPTING A PARTICULAR MOVE. RATHER, YOU'RE FORCED TO FACE YOUR FEARS AS WELL AS YOUR OPPONENT.**

Going Solo

Learning forms is the culmination of having mastered enough of the basics to be able to perform several of them in a sequence by yourself. Learning your first form is like your first solo driving experience. All the in-class and on-the-road instruction come into play as you experience the independence of mastering a complex set of rules and reactions. In this case, your improved strength, stamina, speed, and flexibility pay off, as well as your knowledge of timing, focus, breathing, and balance.

As you learn the steps and techniques of your first form, your background in self-defense techniques will also come in handy. You'll realize that each technique within the form has an application. That scooping motion you make with your hand? That's in response to an imaginary kick—you're scooping it away from you. That two-handed movement that looks showy? It's actually a block and a strike in one.

While forms involve imaginary opponents, sparring involves very real ones. For that reason, it is one of the most contentious aspects of the martial arts, and one that deserves greater coverage than can be given here. Chapter 5 will cover that topic in detail. Suffice it to say that in sparring you'll be expected to work with partners on a level unlike any before. You'll need to size up your partner, strategize on how best to defeat her, and endure lengthy sets without giving up. Indeed, unless you get injured or feel sick, you must spar until the instructor ends the match.

For some students, forms and sparring represent the pinnacle of their training. For others, it goes on to include classical weapons training. While the term "weaponless warrior" is overused, it does accurately sum up how the majority of the arts encompass "empty-handed" fighting techniques. However, it's not completely accurate. Classical weapons play a role in the martial arts, and have for centuries. As a new student, however, you won't be expected to master weapons, and in some schools, you'll never even pick up a weapon.

But somewhere down the line, you may be introduced to weapons, or develop an interest in them on your own. And because classical weapons training complements empty-handed training, it pays to understand some of the more common weapons and how they're used. Four of them are:

Bo. A bo is simply a bamboo pole approxi-mately six feet tall. It was originally used by Okinawan farmers as a substitute for weapons confiscated by invaders. In addition to blocking, the bo is useful for striking and sweeping.

Nunchaku. If you've ever watched a martial arts film, you've probably seen the nunchaku in action. It was originally used to flail grain, but, like the bo, was incorporated into a weapon by farmers. It consists of two sticks of equal size and weight connected at one end with a chain or cord, and is used to whip, block, strike, choke, and pinch.

Sai. The sai, which usually comes in pairs, resembles a thin knife, with a blunt end, about twenty inches long flanked by two opposing prongs running parallel to the knife, but stopping about a third of the way up. It is used to whip, butt, poke, block, and trap.

Tonfa. Originally used as a millstone handle, the tonfa was later used to deliver powerful blocks, thrusts, or strikes. Today, some law-enforcement agencies, realizing its greater versatility, have substituted their nightsticks for tonfas. Tonfas are eighteen inches to twenty-four inches long, made of hard wood, and have a short handle that juts out about one-fourth of the distance from the bottom. It is held by the handle so the shaft runs along the outer forearm.

A Thinking-Woman's Sport

For some nonpractitioners, the martial arts is too regimented. They see students marching to the tune of the instructor. If he tells them to fall to the floor and do twenty push-ups, they do it. If he tells them to throw punches and kicks at one another, they'll do that, too. Rather than developing individuality, the martial arts saps it out of its practitioners, leaving them virtual automatons.

To the uninitiated, it probably appears that way. But what they don't see are the individual touches students bring to their art, as well as the mental benefits that come from sharpening one's concentration and learning to think positively.

The beauty and skill a martial artist brings to a sparring match cannot be wholly appreciated by someone who has never tried it. What isn't readily apparent is the strategy that goes into planning a move. Certainly, the ability to think on your feet isn't only expected, but necessary to avoid injuries.

Developing the ability to strategize allows you to use the most effective technique, while expending the least amount of energy. Adept martial artists are in fact expert decision-makers. Throwing a simple technique is a study in decision-making. What technique to throw? Where to throw it? When to throw it? In fact, the more you study, the more you'll strategize your moves rather than throw random techniques. You'll learn to spar using your mind first, your body second. You'll learn to evade oncoming techniques, fake techniques, and to set up your opponent to practically walk into your moves.

You'll learn when a technique is about to be thrown at you before it's thrown, or when to detect someone coming at you from behind. In my first school, this latter ability was developed by having students stand with their eyes closed as the instructor walked quietly around them. Students would try to detect when the instructor was near them, relying on hearing and sensory perception to guide them. In my current school, the instructor turns off the lights, and pairs of students spar in slow motion. With only the light of the moon shining through the windows to guide us, students sharpen their ability to detect a punch or kick before it touches them.

To sharpen your mind, you need to clear it. That's why many schools spend a few minutes before and after class letting students sit quietly, backs straight, chins tucked in, eyes closed, breathing in through the nose and out through the mouth. I've read about one instructor who has his students visualize themselves floating in cold dark water while a soft current brushes against them. As students try to feel the water, their minds become quieter. Just a couple of minutes of this lowers anxiety levels and improves concentration.

This meditative aspect of the martial arts isn't just a carryover from the days when monks studied them. With all a student must keep in mind when working with a partner or practicing a form, it's imperative that she be free of distractions. That means not thinking about the argument she had with her boss that day, or the driver who tailgated her all the way to class. A wandering mind, especially while working in pairs, leads to injuries and sloppy technique.

While meditating is intended as a calming exercise, some students find it difficult to concentrate while sitting in the traditional leg-numbing position known in Japanese as seiza (SĀYZAH), which means formal sitting. Not only is it used in tea ceremonies and Buddhist services, seiza is also inflicted as a punishment on schoolchildren in Japan. Here's how it works: The spine is kept straight and the legs are folded underneath the body with knees on the ground, the tops of the feet flat on the ground with the soles facing upward and toes pointing backward, and the rump resting on the heels. Martial arts students may sit this way nearly motionless for ten minutes or more. Because it is almost impossible to get up quickly from the position for purposes such as lunging at one's enemy, seiza is considered a sign of respect and attentiveness.

In addition to seated pre- and postclass meditation, martial arts students generally practice a brief standing version of it before and after a form. Though how it's done varies with every style, one way involves beginning a form by inhaling deeply and exhaling loudly, emptying the body of air right before inhaling deeply again and starting the form. The form ends by placing the left hand atop the right hand, bringing them in toward the chest, then down to rest near the groin area—a gesture that represents the student gathering her ki, or energy, then tucking it in her. Like meditation, these gestures enable the student to focus on what she's doing and clear her mind of distractions.

And often there are distractions, such as students, instructors, and perhaps potential students observing class. Getting used to performing forms before a group of onlookers was one of the toughest challenges I faced in the martial arts. That and yelling. Many styles require practitioners to release deep abdominal shouts when executing a technique. It not only unbalances your opponent, but makes your technique more powerful by forcing you to exhale as you implement the technique. Keep this in mind as you attempt to deliver your shout. Your instructor won't allow you to be the sole student who doesn't have to execute such a yell, and holding back only results in a weak screech that will surely draw more attention than if you had put your all into it.

But uttering these deep abdominal shouts isn't the only time you'll be called on to use your voice. Many traditional schools require students to recite their style's history and identify techniques by their English and Asian names. During warm-ups, my instructor often calls on a student to describe how our style of karate developed; during drills, he might call on a student to identify the kick the class is practicing.

Though you never knew when he might call on a student, or what student he would call on, you could always count on being drilled on history and terminology during a promotional test. During my green-belt test, I was asked to name the style of martial art we studied. Obviously, I had let my nerves get the best of me, and couldn't for my life remember the Japanese term. My instructor had the brilliant idea of making me do push-ups until I remembered. It worked. As part of my black-belt test, I was not only quizzed on terminology, but had to submit a ten-page paper describing the history of my style, as well as why I decided to study it.

But history and terminology quizzes are a once-in-a-while occurrence. In traditional schools, students are always expected to adhere to certain formalities. In my school, bowing upon stepping onto, and leaving, the training floor is required, as is thanking a student, in Japanese, for having worked with you on a technique, and verbally acknowledging something the instructor said.

When you add up the physical and mental demands placed on students, you realize why so many practitioners say the martial arts is more a way of life than something you leave behind in class. Certainly, not all schools focus on every training aspect covered here. But many of them do. By understanding what's out there, you'll find it easier to live up to the expectations of your chosen school.

5. Sparring

*I*F I EVER OPEN A karate school, it will concentrate on basics and forms. I might even teach students to perform self-defense techniques based on basic moves. Sparring will be limited to a light, no-contact exercise. Any student caught "accidentally" hitting another student would be subjected to after-school push-ups.

Certainly, many martial arts students envision the "perfect" school where the workouts are tailor-made to their liking. Perhaps that's precisely why there are so many martial arts schools. By the time a student attains a black belt, she no longer feels compelled to follow the teacher's instructions, and decides to open her own school.

But since I have no plans to open a school, I'll continue to train according to the rules set out by my instructor. I'll continue to work one-on-one with a partner, practicing self-defense moves that involve throwing, wrist grabs, head locks, and a wide assortment of awkward positions. And I'll spar. I'll spar slow when the teacher instructs us to spar slow, concentrating on perfecting my blocks, kicks, and punches.

When he gives the command to spar hard and fast, I'll throw strong punches that stop just short of hitting my opponent. I'll summon up loud, forceful abdominal shouts as I execute kicks and punches. But I won't always feel comfortable doing it. Nor will I feel completely safe in this situation.

And I know I'm not alone. Many female karate students express similar feelings about sparring. In fact, some label it the number-one reason women quit the martial arts. Sure, you feel an extraordinary sense of accomplishment after a successful sparring session—you sustained no injuries, you got in a few good techniques, and your strategy for evading your opponent's moves worked. But the desire to crawl off the training floor and never return is the sensation following an unsuccessful session—your partner, apparently unable to grasp the concept of "no contact," hit you in the chest, then proceeded to sweep you, literally, off your feet, sending you landing the floor.

Women's aversion to sparring is reflected in the *Black Belt* magazine survey mentioned in Chapter 1. Of the women surveyed who stopped training, most did so because they disliked sparring. Most of them quit at brown-belt level, when sparring becomes more intense. Some said they would consider resuming training if they could find a school in which sparring was not a major portion of the training.

Some women take to sparring like fish to water. They navigate themselves around their opponents, darting in with quick, deliberate moves, then just as quickly slipping out of harm's way. Chances are these women aren't intimidated by sparring; they may even thrive on the challenge and competition inherent in tournaments. Others, like myself, are content to spar in class, then put away their fighting equipment until the next class.

I've read about women with a lot of pent-up anger, often from abusive childhoods or abusive relationships, who fight with such abandon that their larger male opponents can't keep up. But toning down a student's aggression is probably easier than developing more aggressive behavior. Women who, abused or not, hesitate to throw the first punch, or can't summon up the courage to throw her opponent, require the most encouragement.

In my seven years of training, I've yet to meet a woman who thrives on sparring. I know they exist because I've seen them at tournaments, and read about them in martial arts magazines. Most of the female martial artists I know approach sparring cautiously, not really loving it and not really dreading it. Others do approach it, however, with a sense of dread, consumed with the idea that an injury is just a fist away. Why don't they approach sparring with the enthusiasm they bring to their warm-ups, basic-moves drills, and forms? Why don't they consider themselves lucky to be allowed to move on to a higher form of training?

A great deal of the apprehension women, and men, bring to sparring can be addressed by the instructor. Certainly, the instructor is the one person who can control students and set an example for the class. Unfortunately, it's the rare instructor who addresses women's concerns about sparring. More often than not, he is more inclined to address their concerns after it's almost too late. He's more likely to make concessions when a female student tells him she's leaving his school because she's tired of being injured during sparring matches while the instructor stands by without issuing any warning to her sparring partner.

Certainly, students have limited control over their teachers, and threatening to leave the school works only if the student has been there long enough for the instructor to develop respect for her and the knowledge that by letting her go he's losing a good student. But threats don't serve anyone in the end.

Assuming you use the information provided in Chapter 3 to find a qualified, concerned instructor, I'm convinced you can ease yourself into sparring and learn to enjoy it. By starting early in your training, you'll be able to hone the traits I think are key to enjoying and excelling at sparring. In time, you'll feel less apprehensive about sparring, and may even come to feel the same way about sparring as you do about warm-ups, basics, and forms. From my experience, I'd say there are three key traits to safe, enjoyable sparring:

- attitude
- instinct
- intelligence

Developing a positive attitude can mean the difference between quitting and persevering. Fine-tuning your ability to detect what your opponent has in mind for you helps ensure your protection. And using your mind as much, or more, as your physical abilities will allow you to outsmart the competition. This chapter will expand on these concepts, as well as other aspects of sparring, because the more you know about sparring, the less likely you'll be intimidated by it.

What Is Sparring?

Chances are your instructor will not let you spar until you've attained a certain level of physical fitness and have mastered some basic techniques. That means being able to withstand a hit should you be unfortunate enough to take one. It also means you understand not only how to perform basic punches, kicks, and strikes, but why they are performed the way they are. Once you've progressed that far, you will be slowly introduced to sparring.

One of the best ways for new students to start learning about sparring is by observing it in action. Take every opportunity to carefully watch your classmates spar. It's too easy and common for new students to let their minds wander during a sparring session because they don't understand what's happening. Indeed, to a novice, sparring can look fairly unstructured and disorderly.

Start by comparing sparring to other sports. Sparring is probably most similar to boxing in that the fist is used to strike an opponent. Because of the similarity, you will probably routinely observe some beginning male martial artists boxing with their opponents rather than sparring—something the instructor should be quick to correct. In this instance, a student will come into his opponent with his arms held close to himself, hands protecting his face, then he'll lash out with a series of short jabs to the opponent's face or gut.

> **MARTIAL MAXIM: "AEROBIC BOXING" HAS DEVELOPED AS AN ALTERNATIVE TO BASIC WORKOUTS AMONG WOMEN. IT WILL BE INTERESTING TO SEE WHETHER IT CATCHES ON AND WHETHER IT ATTRACTS MORE WOMEN TO THE MARTIAL ARTS.**

Unlike boxing, sparring involves more numerous and complex techniques. The emphasis here is on executing clean, effective techniques. Only techniques that are thrown correctly count; a sloppy technique, even if it successfully strikes your opponent, would not count. In most cases, you won't actually be hitting your opponent. Light- or no-contact sparring is the norm in most classes; full-contact sparring is usually limited to certain tournaments.

To understand sparring, you need to understand the concept of offensive and defensive. When a student goes on the offensive, she is playing the role of attacker or aggressor. Perhaps part of the reason so many women are turned off by sparring is because the word "offensive" is synonymous with displeasing, rude behavior—a trait most women were taught from an early age not to display. A defensive person, on the other hand, resists aggression. Here, the student would be likely to execute blocks against her opponent's kicks and strikes. Most women I've observed sparring behave defensively during a match. But as we'll see, this strategy can at times be extremely effective.

If accepting that offensive behavior is a necessary part of martial arts fighting is difficult for some women, learning to forfeit control is even tougher. Between the time a student begins training and the time she starts to spar, she has basically been in control. Forms and basic-moves drills certainly give students a great deal of control. In most instances, students performing forms and drills are working by themselves, and any mistakes they make will not cause them to incur a hit from another student. Even self-defense drills enable students to retain control. Though performed with a partner, self-defense drills are usually well-choreographed, with the instructor talking students through every step; hence, these drills also allow students to maintain a high degree of control. On the other hand, sparring introduces into training risk and the unexpected.

Sparring is also a strong reminder to students that they are studying a fighting art. It's important for beginning students to occasionally remind themselves of this. Though obvious, this fact often gets lost on new students who become all-consumed with perfecting basic moves and practicing them in forms. Since the martial arts teaches that no student, even an advanced black belt, can ever attain perfection, many students become intent on coming as close to perfection as possible. But basic moves and forms are not just for show; they serve a practical purpose. As you learn basic blocks and strikes, think about how they might be applied to an opponent and why they are thrown the way they are. If you're not sure, ask the instructor.

Indeed, use your role as new student to begin preparing yourself for sparring. All too often, new students don't give sparring a second thought, then are terrified when they realize their instructors want them to start participating in class sparring. By observing students sparring now, you will be that much less intimidated when it comes your turn to stand facing an opponent in the center of the training floor.

Certainly, you'll have time to observe lots of sparring

matches since it will probably be a while before you're expected to spar. New students will focus solely on rolls, grabs, throws, blocks, punches, strikes, and kicks. During this part of your training, what will quickly become apparent is that basic moves are anything but basic. For example, learning to throw a punch is not as simple as clenching your fist and throwing it out in front of you. You have to understand how to make a fist, what part of the fist strikes the target, how both arms come into play, and what role the hips play.

Later, students are taught to combine basic moves. Again, it's not as simple as it appears, so keep this in mind when frustration sets in. Consider this: If you have ten instructions to think about when throwing a punch, you now have perhaps as many as twenty going on at once as you learn to execute a punch followed by a block. After successfully coordinating two basic moves, you'll learn to perform three, then four, and so on until combining as many as ten moves becomes second nature.

Eventually, students are teamed up with high-ranking partners who help them learn throwing, choking, and holding techniques designed to immobilize an opponent, as well as advanced escape techniques. As new students become more accustomed to working with partners on these self-defense drills, the students develop distance, timing, speed, power, and eye-hand coordination. At each level, from learning the basics to working on self-defense moves with a partner, you should be comparing what you've learned to the students you observe sparring.

When students are comfortable and fairly adept at these training techniques, they are ready to begin sparring on a limited basis. If they are studying karate, tae kwon do, or kung fu, it will be referred to as sparring. If they are studying aikido or judo, it will be referred to as randori. Though they go by different names, the premise is basically the same—to put all the moves learned into practical application in order to conquer an opponent.

You'll often hear aikido referred to as a noncombative martial art because it emphasizes throws and joint techniques over striking and kicking. Here, students learn to move with a push, and if pulled, move with that motion, in effect blending with an opponent's movement and direction of power. However, aikido incorporates randori training just as judo does in which one student is attacked or set upon by one or more students.

Still, aikido is one of the least aggressive martial arts. At the opposite end of the spectrum are styles such as Shukokai karate, where students are taught to move straight into an opponent while throwing a series of rapid-fire punches, strikes, and kicks. These students waste no time in getting to their opponents, and for this reason often excel at point sparring.

Warming Up to Sparring

Students cannot avoid sparring simply by avoiding tournaments. Sparring is as much a part of martial arts training as warm-ups. While there isn't the degree of competition in class as there is in a tournament, the element of competition is still there—and that alone makes some people nervous.

Sparring is by nature competitive—something not everyone feels comfortable with. Whether women are naturally disinclined toward sparring, or whether society encourages women to avoid competition, is subject to debate. Some theorize that because women were for years barred from competitive sparring, they never felt comfortable with it. But there are certainly enough female martial artists today who excel at sparring to dispute this theory. And from observing children's martial arts classes, in which boys and girls routinely spar with one another, I'd say sparring will become less and less of an issue for adult martial artists of the future.

What's certain is that women are capable of enjoying and

excelling at sparring. Again, it goes back to the instructor, and how he approaches it. Does he set up and enforce rules for sparring? I've seen students hit their opponents with full force when the instructor clearly stated no contact. I've seen students grab their opponents by the arm or wrist and attack with their free hand knowing that this wasn't allowed. I've seen students kick their opponent in the kidney when they know better than to strike in such a sensitive area. I've even heard of instructors who use sparring as a punishment, pitting a beginning student against a high-ranking student, then allowing the latter student to attack with full force. If these are the kinds of rules your school follows, find another.

When students don't play by the rules, and instructors don't enforce the rules, injuries usually result. Whether the rules are shunned through malice, ignorance, or the desire to win is irrelevant. What's important to remember is that these types of students exist, and it's up to you to deal with them.

Teachers can only deal with these types of students to an extent. If certain students only occasionally injure other students, the instructor probably won't reprimand them. But that's not reassuring to you. What's important here is that you find an instructor who eases new students into sparring slowly, teaching and reinforcing the rules along the way.

In the school I attend, new students initially just observe other students sparring. As two students spar in the middle of the training floor, new students sit quietly to the side as a high-ranking student explains to them what the sparring students are doing, as well as some of the rules. Later, new students' training will incorporate slow-motion sparring with high-ranking students who instruct the new student when and where to throw and block kicks and punches. Eventually, the pace is increased, and the student isn't told what moves to throw and when to throw them.

As students begin to spar, they rarely incur injuries. That's because instructors are generally extremely careful during this period in the student's training. As training progresses, you'll find that your opponent becomes more aggressive, and unless you do, too, you discover how easy it is to get hit. At this point, the instructor encourages you to defend yourself more, and strategize how to get to your opponent before she gets to you.

> **MARTIAL MAXIM: THOUGH AN INTEGRAL PART OF THE MARTIAL ARTS, SPARRING IS NOT THE PREFERRED WAY TO RESOLVE CONFLICT. THOROUGH MARTIAL ARTS TRAINING INCLUDES AVOIDING VIOLENCE AND SUBDUING AN OPPONENT WITH THE LEAST AMOUNT OF FORCE.**

Ideally, sparring doesn't involve injury. Students stop their techniques just as they touch their opponents. Kicks barely tap an opponent's head. Punches touch an opponent, then quickly withdraw. Opponents go with a throw, landing smoothly on the floor. When it works well, sparring and randori are cooperative give-and-take exercises. Practitioners get to, literally, think on their feet, while enjoying an aerobic workout and strength conditioning.

While many women would prefer becoming accomplished at forms, weapons training, and perhaps teaching, not all schools will let them do this. The only student I've ever heard of who didn't have to spar, but was nevertheless allowed to train at a tae kwon do school, was a grandmother who said she was too old to endure the kinds of injuries common in sparring. Apparently, her teacher agreed.

If you attend class regularly and on time, don't pester your instructor to promote you, and put your all into workouts, your instructor may cut you some slack when it comes to sparring. Maybe he'll team you up with students closer to your weight and height, or with students who spar with caution. Who knows? As your training progresses, you may even look forward to a challenging sparring match.

Types of Sparring

Sparring is either "prearranged" or "free style." In pre-arranged sparring, students are told specifically how to attack or defend themselves. One student might, for example, be told to step forward while throwing a kick to her opponent, followed by a strike to the head. Her opponent, knowing what technique was coming before it was even thrown, would block the kick, then the strike with predetermined techniques. As soon as the attacking student finishes her techniques, she'll become the defender as her opponent throws the same kick and strike.

Prearranged sparring has several variations. One student might step forward with her attack as the defender steps backward, forward, or to the side in order to block the move, then immediately counterattacks. A student may also attack more than once with the same technique while her partner keeps stepping back and blocking the attacks. After the last attack, the opponent counterattacks as many times as her partner did with the same move. A student may also attack with several prearranged techniques as the defender retreats and blocks the attacks. At the end of the attacks, she delivers a forceful counterattack of her own.

Another form of prearranged sparring, but which more closely resembles free-style sparring, has both partners moving around freely. One student attacks with a prearranged technique—a side kick, for example—directed at a pre-arranged target—say, the opponent's head. The defender blocks and counters the attack with the same kick or perhaps a different technique, but one that both students have agreed upon in advance. A more advanced variation of this involves two students who decide who will be the attacker and defender; only the method of attack and choice of weapon remain undisclosed.

Free-style sparring is the most advanced form of training. Here, students are free to throw any technique in any combination as many times as they like. Generally, one student will come in with one, two, or more techniques. If the techniques are successfully blocked, the opponent will generally move into the other student with her own techniques. This back-and-forth exchange in free-style sparring differs from competitive karate in that it is still a method of training whereby students work with each other in perfecting their skills in a realistic situation. When attacks are thrown, they are pulled just short of contact so injury is avoided. Nevertheless, students generally wear protective equipment to avoid taking the impact of an out-of-control technique.

MARTIAL MAXIM: THOUGH THERE ARE SEVERAL TYPES OF SPARRING, ALL CONSIST OF PERIODS OF LOW ACTIVITY INTERSPERSED WITH BRIEF FLURRIES OF DEMANDING, FORCEFUL WORK.

Then there's the ultimate in fighting: free-style, full-contact sparring. Though generally reserved for competitions in tournaments, full-contact sparring is performed in some schools. Of course, as in most sparring, protective head and body equipment is worn, and certain areas of the body are off limits. But that doesn't mean you can't still get injured, and that all students avoid off-limit areas.

Sparring can also be performed with more than one partner, with weapons, and on the ground. In my school, multiple-partner sparring is usually done only with advanced students, and often during a promotional test. Generally, the instructor assigns each attacker a number, then calls the numbers out one at a time. As he does, each student with the corresponding number attacks the defending student. This type of sparring is usually well-supervised, and, surprisingly, few injuries occur. (Only during black-belt tests is the assigning of numbers omitted, and attacking students allowed to attack in any order and more than one at a time.)

Sparring with weapons is also popular. Here, an attacking student comes at her opponent with a fake weapon—a rubber knife, for example. Another form of sparring is ground fighting, which involves the defending student lying on her side on the floor against a standing attacker. The attacker tries to get past her opponent's kicks to get close enough to throw a kick or punch of her own. This type of training prepares students to fight even after they've been knocked or swept to the floor.

Occasionally, my instructor has students practice light-contact, free-style point sparring. Here, the class breaks up into two teams, with one person from each team facing off in the center of the training floor and sparring. A point is scored when one student executes a clean, effective technique. Usually, during each match, a student takes a turn standing across from the instructor to referee. These students are responsible for helping the instructor decide whether a student's technique deserves a point. To add an element of competition, the losing side must do push-ups or drag themselves across the floor using only their arms.

Though an entertaining way to learn about point sparring, this in-class exercise was the closest I wanted to get to competitive karate. I've competed in tournaments, but only in forms. I like to have some control over who I spar. In class, at least I'm familiar with each student's style; at a tournament, even one that doesn't allow full-contact matches, I not only don't know the student, but I don't know the teacher or the school.

In tournament sparring, two students go back and forth until one throws a clean, effective technique. Karate students wear protective equipment, and throw punches, strikes, and kicks within a defined area, usually on a hardwood floor. Choking, head butting, knee and elbow strikes, biting, holding and striking, and striking when an opponent is down are prohibited. In full-contact karate, contestants fight to the knockout. In semicontact karate, light contact is allowed.

In judo, students work on a mat, grasping each other's jackets and trying to throw each other using pins, chokes, and armlocks. The objective is to apply foot techniques designed to unbalance the opponent, timing, and the techniques themselves, with emphasis on posture and form. Amateur karate matches generally consist of three two-minute rounds; judo matches generally run six to ten minutes. (Judo is the only official martial art included in the Olympics, having been adopted in 1961.)

As late as the 1970s, women judoists were restricted to competing in forms. Today, they can compete in randori tournaments. In most cases, the only difference between men's and women's randori is that the women's rounds are shorter. However, women occasionally spar with men, such as when not enough students have signed up to create two separate competitions.

If you attend a sparring competition, you're likely to see a referee standing in the fighting area, a judge seated at each of the four corners of the match area, and one arbitrator seated to one side of the match area. The referee conducts the match, awards points, announces fouls, and issues warnings and disciplinary actions. The judges can override a referee's decision, and help decide in case there is no clear winner. A winner is declared when a contestant has three points or if the match is over and the score is two to zero.

Sparring Tips

If sparring was only about strength, few women would excel at it. It's precisely because sparring involves timing, speed, and intelligence that women can and do excel at it.

Developing timing and speed doesn't happen overnight. Unfortunately, before that happens many new students drop out. It's common for women to quit the first time they have to spar a man twice their size. Or the first time they get thrown or swept to the floor. Or the first time they get hit.

In a way, you can't be afraid to get hit. If you let fear overcome you, your techniques will get sloppy and you'll be more likely to look away, exposing yourself to injury. You've got to learn to build your confidence, and at the same time, learn to trust your partners. But don't trust them to the point where you get injured. I've seen students ignore oncoming techniques because they know their sparring partner can be trusted to stop the technique just before it hits them. These students won't bother to block the technique, and will often go right into a counter technique. This is not sparring.

On the other hand, there will be students who you may never trust. Take these students with a grain of salt. You can't avoid sparring with them, but you can avoid injuring yourself. How? Start by approaching sparring and randori with a confident, positive attitude. If you do, you'll already be ahead of the majority of the students in your school.

Even with the right attitude, you'll still be exposed to risk. But risk is inherent in sparring and randori—and most of life for that matter. The trick is to minimize risk. The following twelve sparring tips are designed to do just that—reduce the risk of injury so you cannot only excel at sparring, but enjoy it.

1. Relax. Most first-time sparrers are visibly tense. Their shoulders are raised to their earlobes, their bodies stiff, and reactions jerky. Their facial expressions border on near-fear.

So how am I supposed to relax if my sparring partner has fists the size of cantaloupes? you might be thinking. A certain amount of tenseness can help your sparring by keeping you alert. Too much, and your moves won't be effective. Try taking a couple of deep breaths before sparring begins, and remember that your partner is probably as, or more, uptight than you.

2. Defensive strategy works. When it comes to in-class sparring, too many new students sustain injuries because they assume they've got to keep throwing techniques. Don't pressure yourself to always be the attacker. Half the battle during in-class sparring is to stop your opponent from hitting you.

To that extent, you'll want to concentrate on blocking your opponent's offensive techniques, then countering them. This evading-and-controlling strategy takes the pressure off you to strategize what to throw, and lets you instead concentrate on protecting yourself. Once you've blocked your opponent's technique, then you can look for an opening to apply your own technique. If that's too aggressive for you, throw one technique for every three or four your opponent throws. There are no rules that say you must throw a technique for every one your opponent throws.

Of course (and you probably saw this one coming), the opposite works extremely well, too. By surprising your opponent with a quick, sudden, offensive attack, you can get a solid technique in before your opponent has begun to think about what technique she'll throw. I've seen students stand stunned as their opponents got in the first technique. Try it after you have some sparring experience under your belt.

3. Avoid putting yourself at risk. Beginning students often don't think about the consequences of their actions. I've seen students walk straight into an oncoming technique, or throw a technique while looking away as if by not seeing her partner's response to it, she won't get injured. Keep an arm's-length distance from your partner unless you're coming in to throw a technique. And never, ever take your eyes off your partner.

Keeping your eyes on your partner begins even before the first technique is thrown. Notice when two partners bow before beginning a sparring match, neither one takes her eyes off the other. This tradition goes back to the days when you couldn't trust your partner not to throw a technique before the match officially began. Certainly, you didn't want to be caught staring at the floor as your partner threw a kick into your face. Today, keeping your eyes on your opponent is done mainly for ceremonial reasons.

4. Keep it simple. Students who excel at sparring more often than not rely on basic techniques. Not only are these types of techniques effective, they're less likely to get you injured. For a karate student, this might mean throwing a simple straight punch instead of a spinning back fist strike. For a judo student, it might mean applying an inner thigh throw instead of a stomach throw, which is impressive but requires superb timing. In fact, some martial artists, such as karate champion Bill "Superfoot" Wallace, have built a career based on one basic technique they use to win numerous matches. (Can you guess what area of the body Wallace favors using?)

Fancy or not, techniques aren't your only weapons. Try faking a technique, say a punch, by throwing it halfway, then withdrawing it and throwing a different technique, say a kick. If your opponent is heavy, he may not be able to adjust quickly enough to block the kick. With this type of opponent, it also pays to move around a lot to tire him out before throwing a technique.

5. Kiai (KEE-Ī). If your style of martial arts allows you to utter those deep abdominal shouts as you throw a technique, then use them. I've seen too many students, and not only women, shy away from using them. But they actually do unnerve your opponent. What's more, it makes your technique stronger by forcing you to exhale at the right time.

6. Keep your mouth closed. Even the best sparrers get injured. But there's no reason to inflict pain on yourself by biting your tongue. That means no lazy tongues hanging out of your mouth or pushing against your teeth as you concentrate on the task at hand. I follow a bit of advice given to me years ago by my orthodontist. He told me to keep my tongue on the roof of my mouth to prevent it from resting on my front teeth and pushing them out. When applied to sparring matches, this advice does wonders for protecting your tongue.

7. Analyze your opponent. Not all opponents are created equal—a situation that works to your advantage. Analyze your partner's height, weight, strength, and even the length of his limbs. If he's a tall judo student, you might want to consider using a one-arm shoulder throw, which is effective against tall opponents. If he's a tall karate student, throwing a kick to his midsection would make more sense than trying to reach his head. If he's heavy, tire him out by never standing in one place too long.

8. If you send signals, make sure they're mixed. The student who stands with her side facing her opponent and her lead foot lightly bouncing off the floor might as well carry a sign that reads, "I'm planning to throw a side kick into you." Likewise, the student who keeps her hand chambered at her side is sending a clear signal to her opponent that she's waiting for the right moment to throw a straight punch with that hand. And chances are the student who stares at her opponent's feet is planning a sweep. It's okay to set up for a throw, a kick, or a sweep, but don't languish in that position long enough to telegraph your thoughts to your opponent.

9. Study your classmates' favorite techniques. It's easy to stare into space daydreaming while two students spar. But just because it's not your turn to spar, doesn't mean you can't be learning something while you're waiting. What you should be doing is analyzing each student for the one or two techniques they consistently throw—and every student favors a certain technique whether or not they know it. As you observe the students in your school spar, make mental notes of the techniques they favor. Then imagine how you would counter them.

If a student favors sweeps and kicks, she'll try to keep her distance from you. To counter this, frustrate her by closing the distance so she can't extend her leg. If she prefers staying in close, throw kicks to keep her away. And if she's accustomed to reacting to one technique, throw several of them in a row to throw off her timing.

In addition to techniques, observe how students react to sparring. Do they move away from an attacking opponent? Then don't be afraid to move into them. Do they wait for their opponent to throw a technique first? Then don't throw it first. Wait for her to throw a technique, then counter. In other words, do whatever it takes to confuse or frustrate your opponent.

Also, take advantage of your opponent's mistakes. If she consistently looks away when throwing a technique, you can almost assuredly counter without being hit.

10. Pay attention to what your instructor says—to an extent. Chances are your instructor will be egging you on to "get closer," "throw harder techniques," or to try that difficult move that gives you so much trouble. Depending on whom you're sparring, you may want to ignore his commands. It's one thing to want to please the instructor, it's quite another to put yourself at risk.

There are some students who are so aggressive and undependable that I keep my distance no matter what. Perhaps they're known to hit hard, or in places most women would prefer not to be hit. I've seen enough women get hit in the chest to know that area of the body isn't as off-limits as a man's groin. In fact, I know some women who would swear that certain male partners actually try to grab their breast during a match. Talk about unnerving your partner! Since you don't have to worry much about being kicked in the groin, your best defense is to keep your hands by your face. In doing so, you'll be protecting your chest area with your forearms.

11. Hide your emotions. This goes back to signaling your next move to your opponent. Avoid it. By hiding and controlling your emotions, you confuse and unsettle your opponent. If you get hit—and it's not serious—stay calm. It will more likely than not surprise your opponent to the point where he'll be put off guard, giving you the opportunity to counter with your own technique.

You're likely to see a lot of emotions in your school—everything from joy at having passed a tough test to anger to crying. I've seen sparring partners become so angry at each other, technique goes out the window, replaced by an all-out rumble. I've seen grown men on the floor with tears in their eyes, victims of direct groin strikes (which, in my experience, are usually executed by men).

12. Don't always think linear. Beginning students have a tendency to move straight into their opponents or retreat backward away from them. The result is either an injury sustained from having walked into an oncoming technique, to an out-of-bounds call from the instructor because a student backed up past the foul line.

Moving forward and backward is fine as long as the moves complement and work with those of your partner. But in addition to back and forth, you might want to think about using circular movements. Step around your opponent. When done quickly, you can get your technique out before your opponent has time to turn around.

6. Dress Code

MAYBE IT'S BECAUSE I spent six years in parochial school that I feel comfortable wearing uniforms. Sure, I, like just about every one of my female classmates, complained about the pleated skirts that added bulk to our midsections, and the old-fashioned ties and vests. Not until I transferred to public school in seventh grade did I come to appreciate that boring plaid uniform. Suddenly, the biggest decision of the day was made at 7:00 A.M., and the wrong decision might cause you to be excluded from those popular cliques that centered around fashion.

As fashion statements, uniforms don't even rate; as the great equalizer, they excel. By relieving the pressure of having to decide what to wear, uniforms allow you to concentrate on more important matters. They help people define one another by what's inside, not what label is on their backs.

That's probably why I never embraced the health club scene. I always felt that what you wore was as or more important as the number of reps you could do. In fact, I sensed a greater amount of competition in these establishments than I did in any martial arts school. Besides, it's hard to believe that women are comfortable working out in skin-tight outfits that shimmy up in all the wrong places and which are constructed of man-made material that doesn't allow the skin to breathe.

Martial arts uniforms are comfortable because they're loose fitting and are constructed of materials that breathe and don't hold perspiration odors. Best yet, unlike my parochial uniform, they hide body areas many of us would rather not draw attention to.

Schools of Style

To the uninitiated, most martial arts uniforms look alike. Not until you've shopped around for one will you discover the subtle and not-so-subtle differences. Not only do they differ from style to style, but even within one style uniforms differ. In karate, for example, the jacket can be styled long or short, depending on the school you attend. Some schools allow students to wear short-sleeved jackets in hot weather, while others mandate long sleeves year round.

Aside from short sleeves, most uniforms aren't designed for varying degrees of weather. You won't, for example, find uniforms with shorts as opposed to long pants. Certainly, there were many classes during which I would have preferred to wear a short-sleeved jacket with shorts. But for the same reason you rarely see air conditioners blasting on a hot day in most martial arts schools, it's done for practical reasons. (Why don't most martial arts schools blast their air conditioning? Cold air constricts muscles, increasing the possibility they might tear. Schools that have air-conditioners usually turn them on only during the hottest days—and then only on low.)

In addition to maintaining tradition, long pants are more practical than shorts. For one, a uniform that covers most of the body enables students to take falls without getting mat burns. Also, by using the uniform to grab hold of, a student executing a throw can control the person she is working with.

Certainly, most students would rather be grabbed by their pant leg than by their flesh.

That's not to say that students don't adjust their uniforms to increase their level of comfort. I got in the habit early in my training of rolling up my sleeves. Some students also roll up their pant legs above their ankles. (Being five-foot-seven, rare is the uniform that ends below my ankles.) My instructor allowed this—yours may not. However, none of these adjustments are allowed in tournaments, where tradition counts as much as ability.

Understanding the kind of uniform specific to a particular style is as important as knowing how to wear it. In judo, practitioners wear gis (pronounced GEES). The standard judo uniform consists of a white jacket that is reinforced and pants—sometimes reinforced at the knees—secured by a colored belt that signifies the wearer's rank. The jacket is made of two layers of cotton material. For strength, double stitches of thick cotton thread are woven through the jacket and cover the entire upper half of the garment and sleeves. From the waistline to the bottom of the jacket, front and back, a small diamond-shaped design is woven into the fabric.

From the bottom of the right side, around the neck and down the left side, runs a lapel approximately two inches wide, stitched to the body of the jacket. This area is referred to as the scarf, and is often used to choke an opponent—sometimes called a scarf hold. Heavy stitching in each armpit prevents the seams from opening or deteriorating from perspiration. A slit of about seven inches up each side frees the hips. The sleeves are loose; you should be able to pinch at least an inch and a half of material between your thumb and forefinger while wearing the jacket.

You generally won't find uniforms made specifically for male or female students. In fact, the only difference between the uniform of a male and female student is that the female is likely to be the only one wearing a T-shirt beneath her jacket.

The low-cut neckline of uniforms and the grappling action that will at times almost pull the jacket right off you makes it essential that women wear T-shirts. But even male students wear T-shirts to absorb sweat and alleviate the abrasiveness of new uniforms and those made from canvas material. T-shirts also alleviate the aggravation a uniform can have on skin that's prone to acne.

The trousers of the uniform are usually made of cotton fabric, and have a drawstring waist. Like the jacket, the pants, too, must fit loosely, with at least two inches between the bottom edge and the leg. The belt, also made of cotton fabric, is about one-and-a-half inches wide and eight or nine feet long. It is wound twice around the waist and tied in a square knot in front, with the ends of equal length from the knot.

When not working on the mat, judo students wear zori, or slippers, made of rubber or straw and held to the feet à la "flip-flops" with a cord between the first and second toes. The idea is to prevent students from dragging dust and dirt onto the mat from their feet. Since judo practitioners spend a great deal of time rolling and falling on mats, it's understandable that they wouldn't want hairballs and dirt staring them in the face.

Most martial arts schools prohibit any form of footwear on the training floor. In judo circles, practitioners consider their karate counterparts somewhat vulgar in the foot hygiene department because the latter walk barefoot on both the training floor and other areas of the school—in effect, dragging unwanted debris into the training area.

Aside from the footwear controversy, karate uniforms have a lot in common with judo uniforms. They're both referred to as gis, are generally white, and use the system of colored belts to signify rank. However, karate gis lack padding and are lighter because pulling and tugging on a partner's uniform isn't as common as in judo.

If a judo uniform resembles a karate uniform, what does a karate uniform resemble? A tae kwon do uniform. Called a tobok, a tae kwon do uniform resembles a karate uniform except the jacket doesn't open. It slips over the head and has a V-neck collar usually in white or black.

Low-ranking aikido students usually wear judo- or karate-like gis. In some schools, black belt students substitute the pants for a wide, flowing black culotte-style called hakama. These pants are designed to hide leg movement and give the illusion of floating. Unlike karate and judo, not all aikido schools utilize the colored-belt system.

In Chinese kung fu, the sam is the traditional uniform. It consists of a jacket and pants, often black. The jacket has a Nehrulike collar, which, like the cuffs, is sometimes white, and fastens from the neck below by five white ties consisting of a knot that slips into a loop. Kung fu students wear rubber-soled shoes made from black canvas and lined with cotton. Instead of stiff cotton belts, practitioners wear different colored silk or satin sashes.

A kendo practitioner wears a jacket called a keikogi. It's similar to a judo jacket, but is worn tucked into the pants. Rather than colored belts, students' grades are denoted by the color of the uniform. A novice wears a white lightweight cotton jacket, often with crisscross black stitching. High-ranking students wear a heavier or handmade quilted uniform, usually black or navy blue. The bottom half of the uniform consists of the hakama pants worn by some advanced aikido students.

As kendo involves the use of swords (really a practice sword consisting of four pieces of bamboo tied together with a piece of leather that forms the handle), protective equipment is standard—as opposed to karate in which it's worn only during sparring exercises. Hands and forearms are protected by long heavy gloves, and the chest is covered by a breastplate held in place by cords fastened around the shoulders. A heavy quilted waistband with a hip and groin protector is also worn. A steel head and face protector covers the head, throat, and shoulders.

Suiting up for kendo will probably set you back further

than suiting up for any other style of martial arts. A chest protector, head and face protector, gloves, and the hip and groin protector can cost more than $400. The pants will be about $50, and the practice sword $25. A complete karate, judo, or tae kwon do uniform will run about $80. The sparring equipment also adds up, but is not required of new students.

Of course, a tai chi chaun uniform will set you back the least. Students who practice this art aren't required to wear formal uniforms or a colored belt. They can wear loose clothing, and have the option of wearing soft shoes or no shoes.

Buying a Uniform

Before you buy a uniform, ask your instructor if there's a specific style he requires. Some instructors are extremely picky about the uniform their students wear—right down to the patch they want sewn on it. These instructors will either sell you the uniform themselves, or direct you to a store that sells the type he wants. Local merchants are often familiar enough with the schools in the area that they will know what uniform you should purchase. They may even be able to tell you the type of patch the instructor requires his students to sew on their uniforms. Though the merchant may even tell you where to sew the patch onto the uniform, double check with your instructor. Judo instructors, for example, usually require students to sew the patch on the right lapel of the jacket, since the left lapel is constantly grasped during workouts.

Jacket styles are fairly standard; the pants portion of the uniform, however, has been updated. Traditional-style pants are held up with a drawstring, which tends to shred and get tangled after many wearings. In addition, when the drawstring gets wet from perspiration, it becomes almost impossible to loosen. After a particularly sweaty session in my school, it was a common sight in the dressing room to observe two students trying to free a fellow student from her pants by grabbing hold of the sides of the pants of the student in distress and pulling until the drawstring gave, resulting in the two rescuers crashing into the walls as the drawstring finally loosened. Uniform manufacturers have addressed this problem by offering pants with Velcro side closures or an elastic waistband, which in some cases also comes with a thin shoestring drawstring. In addition to updating closures, manufacturers have added a rear pocket on some styles, which is probably for holding a mouth guard.

Though martial arts uniforms are meant to be baggy, it doesn't mean one size fits all. In fact, some uniforms come in as many as ten sizes. Most adult uniforms range in size from three, or small, up to eight, or extra large. Therefore, it pays to try a uniform on before buying it, making sure the jacket and pants are loose but not big. In most cases, you can mix sizes. I prefer my jacket to be a size larger than my pants—it's more comfortable and gives the illusion that I have more bulk on top than I actually do. If the merchant won't let you mix sizes, take your business elsewhere. Or buy your uniform from any one of the many mail order houses that advertise in martial arts magazines—most have hassle-free refund policies, but check before placing your order.

In most cases, your uniform will be white, except if your school uses its own color uniform. You do, however, have a choice of 100 percent cotton material or a cotton/polyester blend. All-cotton material is more "breathable" and keeps its shape. It's also more expensive, and more likely to shrink and need ironing than a cotton/poly blend. I prefer a 100 percent cotton "canvas" uniform because it retains a crispness that adds "snap" to kicks and punches. To avoid ironing and shrinkage, I hang it dry. The result is a stiff, cardboardlike uniform that practically stands by itself. Though it's not for everyone, to me, it felt like I was putting on a crisp new uniform every time, and as a bonus it added bulk to my sticklike figure.

Also, don't worry about the low cut of the jacket's neckline. Wearing a T-shirt beneath your uniform will address that obstacle. Another essential for women martial artists is a sports bra. Not only is breast pain common during menstruation, it is a common problem for many athletic women. A Utah State University study found that 60 percent of female exercisers experienced breast discomfort during or upon completion of their activity. For that reason, an everyday bra isn't as durable as a sports bra and won't give you the support you'll need.

When shopping for a sports bra, splurge and buy one that has a good deal of support. Studies have found that for A- and B-cup women, the common stretchy compression style is fine. For larger-breasted women, a stronger-knit compression bra, an encapsulation bra (which separates your breasts into two cups like a regular bra), or a combination of both works best. Considering that you may be working out in bare feet, which means no sneakers to cushion the space between you and the hardwood floor, you'll need all the support you can get.

MARTIAL MAXIM: A SPORTS BRA IS ONE OF THE MOST IMPORTANT PIECES OF CLOTHING A FEMALE MARTIAL ARTIST CAN OWN.

Before we leave this section, a final word on T-shirts. More women are opting to wear only a sports bra beneath their uniforms. Others wear just a leotard and no bra. Still others are more comfortable wearing a T-shirt with the collar and sleeves cut off. Though you're welcome to wear whatever your instructor allows, keep in mind that in some schools the instructor may ask students to remove their jackets during practice drills so he can correct mistakes hidden by the jacket, including raised shoulders, stiff hips, and bent elbows. It's a common drill in my school for the students to remove their jackets before performing punches and blocks in front of a mirror. Therefore, wear something in which you'll not only feel comfortable, but won't be embarrassed to be seen working out in.

Belt It

What would the martial arts be without belts—those wide strips of cloth wrapped twice around a student's waist and tied in a tight slip knot? Chances are it would take more effort to sum up your proficiency in the martial arts. Certainly, it's a lot easier—and impressive—to say, "Oh, by the way, I just earned my brown belt in karate" than it is to say, "Oh, by the way, I just learned kururunfa kata, which pretty much means I'm a hot shot in martial arts circles."

In Japan, the grading system is less structured, and doesn't include the different colored belts found in the United States and Europe. Legend holds that in the martial art's infancy, students trained outdoors in white uniforms tied with white belts. Eventually, both articles of clothing became soiled and dirty from falls and rolls taken; however, only the uniforms were washed. The belt became brown, then black—hence the black belt.

Not until the martial arts spread outside the Orient did schools adopt a more varied ranking system. By changing belts every six months or so, students' interest was kept high. It also enabled instructors to earn extra money by charging students not only for the belt but the test as well. Gradually, more martial arts instructors began not only teaching their style of martial arts the way they wanted, but adopting their own ranking systems; hence the wide disparities between ranks found even among schools that profess to teach the same style. However, the order of colors—from lighter to darker as the student progresses—remains a common throwback to earlier martial arts days.

Judo and karate use similar ranking systems. Both divide rank into two classes: everything below black belt, and everything above it. Anything below a black belt is considered "kyu" grades. (Kyu, pronounced KĪŪ, means "class.") Black-belt rank is referred to as "dan," pronounced DON).

Traditional judo has five levels of ranks. After training for a short time, students attain fifth kyu. Then they attain fourth kyu. Up until now judo students would wear white belts. During the next three ranks—third, second, and first kyu—students wear brown belts. After training for at least three years, they would earn their first-degree black belt.

But just as the kyu grades work backward—from fifth to first—black belt ranking goes forward, so when you earn your first black belt, you're referred to as "first dan." From first to fifth dan, students still wear black belts. As they progress, from sixth to eighth dan, they can wear a red-and-white belt or a black belt; from ninth to eleventh dan, an all-red belt or a black belt; and at twelfth dan, a double-width white belt or a black belt. This highest rank is called shidan, meaning master grade, and no one has ever held this rank except the founder of judo himself, Kano Jigoro.

In the United States and Europe the judo ranking system is, naturally, more colorful than the traditional judo system. Instead of keeping one belt throughout grade levels, many schools start students with a white belt, then use a yellow belt for the fifth rank; a green or orange belt for the fourth rank; a green or brown belt for the third rank; a brown or blue belt for the second rank; and a brown belt for the first rank.

Prior to 1976, women judo practitioners competing in national competitions were, regardless of their rank, required to wear belts with white stripes running down the middle; men wore only solid-colored belts. Considered unfair and sexist by many in the judo community, this practice was stopped as a result of protests by women who, in defiance of the rule, fought in competitions wearing, regardless of their rank, only white belts. Eventually, as a result of their actions, the ruling was changed.

Though it varies from style to style, karate generally has ten levels of ranking versus judo's five. But like judo, karate's system runs backward for students below black-belt ranking. So a new student would start at a tenth grade and wear a white belt. She'd progress on to ninth grade and so on until she reached first grade. Rather than have a different-colored belt for every grade, many schools use a "tab" system in which the ends of students' belts are wrapped with tabs, which in many cases are just strips of colored electrical tape. Students usually advance from white belt to green to brown before attaining black. Other systems use blue, orange, and purple belts. The tab is always the color of the following belt; so a white belt could earn a yellow tab, a yellow belt a green tab, and so on.

Unlike judo, karate systems are not all the same. Some karate schools don't utilize all ten grades; some use as few as five. Like judo schools, karate schools don't all use the same colored belts. Low-ranking students wear belts ranging in colors from white to yellow or orange to purple, blue, green, and brown.

Aikido also uses the kyu and dan ranking systems, with students starting from fifth or sixth kyu and working their way down to first kyu. Instead of kyu ranks, the tae kwon do rank for students below black belt is referred to as "gup." Students start with white belts, then move to gold, green, blue, red or brown, and black, respectively. Black-belt ranks are called dan.

As martial arts belts are perhaps the most noticeable part of a uniform, it pays to understand how they relate to the rest of the attire. Like blue jeans before there was such a thing as stone-washed denim, martial arts belts start out clean, stiff, and bright. As students train, their belts lose their stiffness, get dirty, fade, and start shredding. Unlike uniforms, however, belts are never, ever washed. More likely than not, you'll earn a new belt before the old one falls apart—if you don't, it's time to sit down with your instructor and discuss your progress, or lack of. Black-belt students generally wear their belts until they feel it's time for a new one. That could mean once it starts showing any signs of age—it starts to fade or lose its stiffness or its deep black color. It could also mean once it turns white and frayed beyond recognition. To these students, their black belt is like an old pair of jeans—it becomes such a part of you that it's difficult to part with, and the more it frays and fades, the better they like it.

On a More Personal Level

One on the most vivid memories I have from my first martial arts school is when one night two new students began. The women were being introduced to the class by the instructor. The new students wore crisp white uniforms. They also sported big hair, heavy makeup, and inch-long fire-engine-red fingernails. I never did catch their names, but I remember the class staring in disbelief at the women's fingernails, probably thinking the same thoughts that were running through my mind: "If we practice any technique involving the face, one of those women will accidentally rip the eyes right out of my head." Fortunately for us and the women, they didn't return for a second class.

Most martial arts schools have strict rules on jewelry, hair clips, and nail care precisely because the injuries they can cause are highly preventable. A necklace can get caught on a mat or a student, and can even choke its wearer; bracelets can be ripped off arms and earrings off ears; rings can cut or bruise other students.

Hair combs and hard or metallic clips can be ripped off or

can puncture the skin if the wearer rolls on them. The best option is to hold your hair back with a soft tie. If you can't do that, try an athletic headband. It keeps hair out of the face, and absorbs the perspiration that would otherwise fall in your face—and if you've ever had sweat combined with mousse or hair spray in your eyes, you know it stings. Some schools permit students to bring onto the training floor a towel to wipe away perspiration. These schools would prefer that students not flick their sweat onto other students or wipe their sweat on their uniforms. When the towels are not being used, they are folded neatly to the side of the training floor. Schools that don't use the towel system will often stop class so one or two students can push mops quickly over the floor to soak up the sweat. A floor that is allowed to remain wet is not only unsanitary, but an open invitation for students to hurt themselves from slips and falls.

No matter how you fix your hair, keep in mind that instructors have little patience with students who fuss with it during class. I've seen female students do everything from play with their hair while the instructor explains a move to fixing it during drills performed in front of a mirror. Most instructors I've seen don't even want students to wipe the sweat from their brow because it distracts from the class's concentration. Imagine how an instructor would react to you adjusting your hair while he's teaching.

Some female students attempt to control their hair with an inordinate amount of hair spray. I recall several times as the women's dressing room filled with a sticky, smelly mist as some inconsiderate student encircled her head with a can of hissing hair spray. Not only did these women annoy and inconvenience their female counterparts, but coming into close contact on the floor with them was no joy either.

I've always worn my nails short, so complying with my school's rules on nail care has never been a problem. But for many female martial artists it is. Long fingernails or toenails can be a hazard to students—and male students are the first to point this out, especially when they've had their wrist grabbed by someone with long fingernails. But even long toenails are a hazard. I know a student who incurred a cut in his mouth when someone with long toenails threw a roundhouse kick that came in contact with his gums. Not only does this rate high on the scale of disgusting injuries, it could have caused all sorts of infections. In addition, students with long fingernails are at risk of having them pushed back or torn off if a partner should suddenly pull away from a grip.

Nail polish, to my knowledge, is generally allowed. It can't hurt anyone, unless its wearer could figure out a way to use it to distract her partner long enough to deliver a winning blow—and to my understanding this has never happened. As with nail polish, makeup is generally allowed, although probably because most instructors are too embarrassed to tell their students they'd prefer they didn't wear it. Like perfume, makeup is all right if worn in moderation.

Therefore, even if you are free to wear makeup, keep it to a minimum. Even waterproof makeup has a tendency to smear on other students' uniforms. I've seen male students with lipstick, rogue, and foundation on the backs of their uniforms—something I'm sure they're not too pleased to find when they take them off. The only makeup I wear to class is a light foundation because I put it on in the morning before work and don't take it off until I wash my face at night. Before I take class, however, I wipe my face with a tissue to remove it as well as any oils that have built up during the day. But even the small amount of makeup that's left eventually stains the collar of my uniform, and rarely comes out in the wash.

This is not to say that the only way you can thrive in the martial arts is by reducing your fingernails to stubs, going makeup-less, and growing your hair long enough so it can be neatly tied back with a soft band. But there is one area in which there is no room for compromise: personal cleanliness.

Chances are you will occasionally find yourself working with a partner whose personal hygiene standards are lower than yours. Body odor can be a powerful weapon against an opponent, but it's no reason to have to endure it. Whether from an individual or his or her unwashed uniform, body odor—and even too much cologne or perfume—can cause you to lose all concentration and thus increase your chance of injury. While you probably don't have to wash your uniform after each class, some people do. I wash my uniform after two or three wears, but change to a fresh T-shirt for every class.

As for oral hygiene, the time to think about your breath is prior to class. Bring along a toothbrush and toothpaste if you're unable to brush at home before class. Standing toe to toe with a partner isn't the time to start worrying about your breath, and for obvious safety reasons, chewing gum or sucking on a breath mint are grounds for pulling you off the training floor. Indeed, the only object in your mouth should be a mouth guard if you're sparring.

Also, before class, don't load up with a heavy meal. If you don't have time to eat a meal and digest it before class, opt for a banana with peanut butter and a glass of milk, or a salad. You can eat after class. But most likely you won't have a big appetite after your workout, which is ideal for those who want to lose weight. You're better off drinking water or juice after your workout to replenish bodily fluids that will more than likely flow freely from your pores. (I've yet to find an exercise that makes me sweat as much as karate.) Go to the bathroom before class. While you can leave the floor by raising your hand and asking the instructor permission, it's rather embarrassing.

Certainly, don't drink liquor before class. Even a small glass of wine can impair your judgment and coordination, causing you to perhaps injure your partner. Moreover, you don't want alcohol surging through your veins as your heart is racing.

It's not necessary to refrain from class during your menstrual cycle. I probably used it more as an excuse for times I didn't feel like attending class than as a legitimate reason for missing class. When I did attend class during my period, I just about always felt better afterward—no cramps or bloating. But women experience their periods differently. If your cramps are so severe that you know you'll have difficulty focusing on what you're doing, skip class. If your period is more of an inconvenience than a painful monthly experience, go to class. The hour or so of hard work will be worth the reward of feeling normal afterward.

For some women, the worst part about attending class during their period is the fear of staining. Certainly, take the time to freshen yourself prior to class. But also ask your female partners to alert you should they see any sign of it during class.

Protect Yourself

To see a picture of samurai warriors in full battle dress is to wonder how they ever got on their horses, or kept from laughing themselves silly just looking at the comical helmets perched atop their heads. Except for the part of the face below the eyes, every body part was more or less covered by layers of woven cloth or metal. Helmets resembled everything from an upside-down Bunt-cake pan to a dunce cap with a chin strap. Their weapon of choice was a sword or bow and arrow, both of which appear difficult to hold.

Then there were the peasants, who could nil afford such elaborate protective equipment. But rather than give up the fight, so to speak, they adapted a less pretentious strategy. Instead of arrows, they carried farm tools. Instead of armor, they stuck with their basic work attire—a shirt and slacks. Though unassuming, these "bare-handed" fighters were forces to be reckoned with.

As a sport, martial arts fighting is limited to the training floor. You don't have to worry about fellow students lurking in the parking lot waiting to attack you, or preparing to shoot an arrow through your heart. Nevertheless, even on the floor, you can get hurt. And while it's possible to take a misdirected or miscalculated punch in the stomach during basic training drills, students are more likely to incur a punch or kick during sparring exercises, which is why most martial arts styles require students to wear protective equipment only when they spar. (Unless, of course, you're studying the swordsman-ship skills found in kendo, in which case you'll wear headgear and breastplates during most of your training.)

When I first started training, much of the protective equipment that's mandatory today was optional then. If I didn't want to wear a helmet, I didn't have to. But sky-high insurance premiums pretty much put an end to that. Today, instructors require their students to wear more equipment. When I started studying the martial arts, students sparred wearing gloves and footpads, also known as boots. Now gear-ing up for sparring requires not only gloves and footpads, but headgear and a mouth guard. Optional are such protective items as forearm and elbow pads, knee, shin and instep pads, rib pads, and chest or breast protectors. There's even a female version of men's athletic supporter and cup, which to my knowledge is optional at most schools. However, it may not be long before more optional items become mandatory.

If all this sounds like a lot of equipment, that's because it is. Fortunately, thoughtful design and lightweight materials make, for the most part, for equipment that's comfortable. As your training progresses, you'll decide what equipment feels right for you. For example, the only time I wore a rib protector was the period prior to and during my black belt test when the amount and forcefulness of sparring was at an all-time high. Then I needed the protection, but quite frankly it felt as though I was wearing what I can only imagine it must feel like to wear a corset. To alleviate the constrictive feeling brought on by the rib protector, I took a pair of scissors to it, cutting off the bottom half, which exposed my stomach but still protected my ribs. I figured I'd rather have the wind knocked out of me from a gut punch, than a broken or cracked rib.

As a new student, you won't be required to buy all the equipment you'll ever need. Initially, you'll only have to carry your uniform to class, since most students prefer to change at the school and some schools don't allow students to wear their uniforms in public except in cases when students perform in tournaments. But as you continue to train, you'll build your equipment collection and find yourself toting a lot of items back and forth to class. And since in most cases you won't know ahead of time whether you'll need your protective equipment, it's a good idea to always have it with you. That's why it pays to invest in a large enough bag to accommodate all the belongings you'll eventually need. Choose one with pockets to hold small items such as your mouth guard, spare tampons, a hair tie, and Band-Aids.

While few would argue that some amount of equipment is essential, some claim that too much equipment makes students poor sparrers. The thinking goes that if I'm protected head to toe with equipment, I don't care if I get hit. Theoretically, my defensive moves—blocks, for example—will suffer as I concentrate only on offensive moves such as kicks and punches.

In addition, equipment often gives students a false sense of security. When you see disclaimers such as "User assumes risk of injury" printed across a rib protector, it means it's possible you could incur an injury to the very area the equipment is designed to protect—and if you do, you can't force the manufacturer to pay your medical bills. The same goes for other types of equipment. Just because you're wearing gloves and foot pads doesn't mean you can't break or jam a finger or toe. Simply put, all the equipment in the world won't protect you 100 percent; it'll only decrease the risk of injury.

Nevertheless, just as you have a degree of choice when it comes to choosing a uniform, you also have some choice when it comes to deciding on protective equipment. Use this freedom of choice, and you'll find yourself enjoying your training a whole lot more.

7. Back to Basics

WITH THE HEALTH AND FITNESS craze entering its second decade, many of us have become so informed as to the hundreds of theories designed to help us lose weight, feel better, and live longer that in our zeal to attain these goals, we overlook some basic fitness tenets. Indeed, in the glamour of infomercials and celebrity endorsements that saturates much of what we watch and read, we forget that staying healthy and fit starts and ends with basics.

But we're taught to jump on the fast track to good health and, we're told, if we run hard enough we'll reach our goals. When we don't obtain the kind of results we're taught to expect, we stop. Perhaps it's this disillusionment with our inability to reap rapid results that's triggering the current backlash to the health and fitness craze.

The martial arts isn't a fast track to anything. The fact that it's a slow, sometimes grueling, often tedious process has been both a boon and a bust for the sport. On the one hand, the strong reliance on martial arts tradition coupled with the almost maniacal importance placed on basic moves do lead to giant leaps in terms of self-discovery and self-improvement. On the other hand, we've been taught to be impatient, and anything that doesn't come quickly is often thought of as not being worth the wait.

Certainly, some students don't care if the martial art they

chose to study is of Japanese or Chinese origin. Some also probably aren't convinced that practicing basic blocks, strikes, and kicks over and over again is the key to advancement. But that's what the martial arts are all about. Boiled down, most martial arts are nothing more than basics with movement, a series of simple moves strung together to create lively, intriguing, effective techniques.

Contrary to what some students might believe, the martial arts have come a long way in terms of adapting to an impatient twentieth century. Admittedly, much of the change has occurred only within the past few decades, such as female judoists being allowed to achieve the same rank as their male counterparts. Moreover, upon joining a school, you won't be required, as you might have been decades—and certainly centuries—ago, to sweep the floor for a year before the master deems you worthy enough to be taught to form a fist.

What you will be expected to do is adhere to certain traditions: Bowing to and thanking students after working with them; removing your shoes before stepping onto the training floor; and refraining from talking on the floor. You'll also be expected to practice basic techniques as long as you study a martial art.

Finally, you will be expected to progress according to the instructor's timetable, which as we've seen earlier can vary tremendously from school to school. Some instructors may slow the progress of students who after several months still can't form a tight fist, or correctly demonstrate a block, or execute a proper kick; some teachers look the other way, promoting slow learners for fear of losing them if they're not promoted. But it's those schools that expect the best from their students—and seem to have all the time in the world to wait for it—that you want to seek out. Those are the high-standards schools that still hold firmly on to enough of the traditions and basics of the arts to maintain their power, purity, and popularity.

MARTIAL MAXIM: THE SLOW, STEADY PACE AND VARIED CURRICULUM FOUND IN MOST MARTIAL ARTS SCHOOLS ARE CONSISTENT WITH RECENT STUDIES THAT SHOW GREATER HEALTH BENEFITS FROM MODERATE, CONSISTENT EXERCISE RATHER THAN INTENSE, SPORADIC EXERCISE.

This adherence to the basics, as well as to levels of tradition that today's students find acceptable, has become the hallmarks of the martial arts. In fact, they have become such an accepted, integral part of most styles of martial arts that few outside the arts recognize them as the important building blocks that they are. Instead, many focus exclusively on the mystical aspects of the arts or on their violent aspects—both of which are reinforced by Hollywood as well as many martial arts instructors themselves as being the core of the martial arts.

But when you strip away these most-talked about aspects of the martial arts, you discover a simple kernel of truth: By placing a high value on tradition and basics, the martial arts have retained their effectiveness and popularity. The insistence that students uphold certain centuries-old traditions and perform over and over again basic grabs, takedowns, blocks, strikes, punches, and kicks is what drives many students to be black belts and others right out the door. Indeed, as you observe a class in action, notice which students seem fixated on every nuance of their moves, while others wear a why-are-we-doing-this-again look of distraught and boredom. Guess which students will thrive in the martial arts and which ones will quit.

Stretching Your Limits

When talking about martial arts basics, it's necessary to discuss the two essential elements that set the stage for maintaining interest in them and excelling at them, namely flexibility and strength. For women, what's especially important to remember is that to excel in the martial arts, you don't have to be a human rubber band or a female version of The Terminator.

Certainly, developing flexibility and strength is important to your basics training. The stronger your techniques, the cleaner they'll look. The more flexible your legs, for instance, the lower your stances will be and thus the more attractive your forms will be. (Of course, not all martial arts styles stress low stances, but as we'll see later in this chapter flexibility also prevents injuries.)

The key to enjoying your training is to determine the level of flexibility and strength you're capable of, and comfortable with, attaining. For instance, no matter how much I train, I still can't do a full split—and truthfully, I'm not particularly interested in attaining that ability. I can't even lean forward to touch my toes without bending my knees, much less put my palms to the floor as several of my classmates can. And no matter how many push-ups I do (and I can't do many), bulk is not what comes to my mind when I pose my biceps before the bathroom mirror.

A certain level of flexibility is, however, essential to the martial arts for three reasons:

- It helps prevent injuries by decreasing the tension on muscles;
- it reduces muscle soreness; and
- it will make your moves more dramatic, and in most martial arts styles, aesthetics, or how your moves look, count as much as effectiveness, or what your moves are intended to achieve.

The way to increase your level of flexibility is through warm-ups and stretching, which almost seem to be the same thing, but are not. Warm-ups raise the temperature of your muscles, decreasing the chance they'll be stressed and injured, and increasing their responsiveness, as well as the blood flow to the muscles. Warming up for martial arts practice is particularly important because many of the moves involve changing direction quickly, which can aggravate and tear tight muscles.

How do you know when you're warmed up? You'll actually feel warm, and your muscles will feel relaxed. And, as explained in Chapter 3, a good warm-up session will increase your motivation. Walking is a great warm-up, but you probably won't have room enough in your school to do it. I've found that a great way to warm up is by jumping lightly up and down in one place, twisting the lower half of my body while keeping my arms bent as though I was running. Even jumping jacks are a great way to warm up.

Once students are warmed up, they can begin stretching. Done slowly and deliberately, stretching promotes flexibility. Before a workout, it reduces your chances of being injured; after a workout, it'll relax your muscles and reduce muscle soreness. A good instructor always ends a class with stretching, especially after a particularly tough session. That's because he knows that after vigorous exercise, students' muscles will be slightly injured. If left alone, the muscles will gradually shorten and tighten with time, limiting flexibility and increasing the chances of injuring the muscles. Stretching after a workout enables students to maintain their flexibility. Instructors also understand that not only is stretching good for students, it's good for business. After all, students with pulled muscles may not work out, and with no students there's no school.

Stretching properly to avoid pulled muscles requires a little time and patience. You should also remember to:

- Hold still while stretching (in other words, don't bounce).

- Hold each stretch for at least fifteen seconds, and preferably for thirty seconds.
- Stop as soon as you feel pain. At that point your muscle
  is telling you that it may be about to tear.

A torn muscle is just that—a muscle whose fibers have
been torn apart. Ideally, you want your muscles to be able to
contract and stretch without tearing. Muscles that aren't
stretched and warmed up will stay contracted most of the
time. If they are then forcibly stretched beyond their limit,
they will tear. In addition to warming up and stretching, new
students shouldn't lose sight of the importance of learning to
relax their muscles to prevent them from tearing. This is why
breathing exercises prior to class are so important.

Unfortunately, even among many fitness-conscious
enthusiasts, stretching out before working out is given short
shrift. They're either too busy, or in their zeal to get their
workout over with, they sprint over the gym's warm-up mats
and land in the Lifecycle seat eager to pedal their way to good
health.

Even at my local YMCA, there are only two mats
available for stretching, and they're tucked away neatly and
unobtrusively in two corners of the room in such a way that
you can enter the room and never see them unless you turn
your head sharply to the right or left. About half the people,
upon entering the room, head straight for the machines.

But ten minutes of stretching can save days of discomfort.
In fact, after you get into the habit of stretching, you'll gain a
renewed appreciation for those who practice the stretching art
of yoga, which is far from the lightweight workout many
associate with it. (Who knows? You might even decide to
supplement your martial arts training by practicing yoga in a
group setting or at home on your own.)

The secret to stretching is time. The more you give it, the
more you'll get out of it. Even though most martial arts

schools will begin every class with warm-ups followed by stretching, it pays to fill the time prior to the official start of class with your own warm-ups and stretches. (And chances are you'll arrive early for class, since most instructors, unless given a good reason, expect their students to be punctual.)

MARTIAL MAXIM: EXERCISE PHYSIOLOGISTS SAY THAT NEARLY EVERY ADULT CAN BENEFIT FROM DOING AS LITTLE AS FIVE TO TEN MINUTES OF STRETCHING AND STRENGTH TRAINING TWO OR THREE TIMES A WEEK.

It's not easy to get yourself into this routine. More often than not, the period prior to the official start of class looks something like this: Students mill around the training floor either staring into space or, if they can get away with it, talking with their fellow classmates. Then there are the students who make themselves comfortable on the floor and halfheartedly stretch out. They might make feeble attempts to touch their toes, or they might lie on their back and try to stretch their back thigh muscles by raising their legs, one at a time, toward the ceiling while pulling them toward their head. While these exercises are common and effective, they've got to be done with effort. In an effort to get the most out of their stretches, some students stretch only from a standing position, thus resisting the lure of the floor.

What also stops students from warming up before class is the idea that they might overexert themselves. You'll see this a lot, even during class—a general reluctance by students to push themselves for fear that they'll be too tired to make it through class or they won't perform up to their potential because they wore themselves out earlier. Don't let yourself fall into this trap. For one thing, you won't overexert yourself doing warm-ups and stretching exercises; you'll only invigorate yourself. Also, a good instructor keeps his finger on the pulse of the class and knows when it has been overworked.

Admittedly, it's difficult to discipline yourself to warm up and stretch out, especially after you begin learning blocks, strikes, kicks, and other techniques pertinent to your style. Your first inclination when you get on the floor will be to practice those moves. But they'll feel and look a lot better if you warm up and stretch out beforehand. The best way I've found to discipline myself to thoroughly warm up and stretch out is to start—where else?—at the top. Here are some top-down suggestions:

Neck: Warm up with neck rolls, slowly rolling one way, then the other. Then stretch your neck muscles by turning your head side to side, and then by touching your right ear to your right shoulder and vice versa. Finally, point your chin up and down.

Shoulders: Warm up by rotating your shoulders forward and then backward. Then, with your hands clenched behind your head, pull one arm until your elbow is pointing toward the ceiling. Then switch to the other arm. Now, lock your hands behind your back and raise them while bending over.

Arms: Warm up by rotating your arms forward, then backward. Now rotate your wrists forward, then backward. Stretch your wrists by bending your fingers backward toward the top of your wrist. Hold one hand up with the palm facing your chest, go around the back of the hand with the other hand, grab the meaty part of the hand, which is located just beneath the thumb, then twist the hand until the palm points sideways. Repeat with the other hand. Next, hold your arms out in front of you with your hands made into fists, then shoot your fingers straight out. Repeat this as many times as you can.

Torso: Warm up by placing your hands on your hips, then rotate your hips clockwise, then counterclockwise. To stretch, push one hip to the right side, then to the left.

Legs: There's nothing worse than sore leg muscles because they're probably the most-used muscles in the martial arts. Standing with feet shoulder-width apart, bend over and, without bouncing, reach for your toes. Hold for at least fifteen seconds, and repeat ten times. Then stand with one side of you facing a wall, placing one hand on it for support. Bend your leg, pull it to your chest, and hold. Then swing it to the side, keeping it bent as if you were going to throw a kick. But instead, grab your shin, pull it toward your body, and hold. Finally, grab your ankle and hold the bent leg behind you. Switch sides and do this with the other leg.

Some of the best leg stretches are done with a partner. With one person standing with her back against a wall, the other student slowly lifts her partner's leg, stopping intermittently to allow the muscle to stretch. The leg is then lowered slowly back down. You can also do this exercise with the leg being lifted to the side.

Feet: Yes, even these need to be warmed up and stretched. Standing with feet shoulder-width apart and hands on hips, rock back and forth on your feet (this also stretches the shin muscles). After that, rotate your foot at the ankle. Then point it up and down. Do the same for the other foot.

At this point in your training, you needn't concern yourself with other students' stretching techniques—unless, that is, you have a question, which you can bring to a high-ranking student. Occasionally, a high-ranking student will approach you to help with your stretches or to show you how to stretch properly. This is how a well-run school operates: High-ranking students assist low-ranking students, constructive criticism is offered, and no one is made to feel inferior. So don't rush through your stretching exercises or push yourself to the point of pulled muscles. Go slow, don't bounce as you stretch, and pay attention to all your muscles, even the ones we haven't specifically gone over.

If you do pull a muscle, or incur some other minor injury, tell your instructor. He should advise you to avoid stressing the muscle until it has healed. If you injure your wrist, for example, you might do sit-ups while the rest of the class does push-ups. If it's your knee that's injured, you might do side bends when the rest of the class is instructed to do knee bends. In any case, don't try to ignore an injury out of fear of being branded a difficult student. In the same vein, if you have a bad back or sensitive knees, avoid stressing these areas. Chances are you're studying a martial art for pleasure and enjoyment, not to prove that you have a high threshold for pain.

Strong-Arm Tactics

Once you've set the stage for fortifying yourself against pulled muscles, you're ready to build strength—a slow, steady process that seems to happen without you even realizing it. In class you may feel like a weakling despite the fact that you do push-ups and other strength-building exercises. But it's probably not until you're outside class that you'll realize the progress you've made. The realization might hit you when you effortlessly open a new jar of peanut butter on the first try. I realized the extent of my strength when, walking along the beach with my parents, I grabbed my mother's hand to help her over a sandbank and practically threw her over it.

As long as you continue to train, your strength will always be there. However, when you stop exercising, your muscles will start to shrink, and you'll lose a degree of strength and endurance. According to one exercise physiologist, if you're in shape, you won't start seeing serious declines for as long as three to six weeks. So don't be excessive with your training. Certainly, you don't have to train every day. It's also probably not a good idea to attend class three days in a row, then stop for the rest of the week. Instead, try spreading your workouts throughout the week.

How do you know if you're training too hard? Physical or mental burnout is the price, according to exercise physiologists. The warning signs of overtraining are fatigue even when you're not working out, susceptibility to illness, a general feeling of staleness, and disrupted sleep. The cure is to take a few days off from exercise.

Even if you do maintain a steady class attendance—say, three times a week: Monday, Wednesday, and Saturday— you may not always feel in top shape. Sure, some days you'll feel superhuman. But other days you'll feel as though your muscles are atrophying. It may have to do with women's menstrual cycle and their body chemistry in general. Though "experts" say athletic performance is not altered by the menstrual cycle, I can't say that I agree. I always feel weakest a day or so before I get my period. It's then that my muscles feel heavy as lead. Other women say they feel weak during their period—a very real physical condition contributed to by the fact that iron is lost in the menstrual blood. But as we've heard hundreds of times, working out before and during your period relieves cramps for most women. So unless you're doubled over in pain, push yourself to attend class during this time.

Even as you begin to feel stronger, keep in mind that to increase strength, you've got to overload your muscles—that is, work them to the point where they begin to hurt. If you continue to do the same number of push-ups week after week, you won't get stronger. You have to push yourself to do more. One reason most students become stronger when they take up a martial art is because they have an instructor who encourages them. Strength training on your own is difficult if only because most of us don't have the discipline, or for that matter personal trainers breathing down our necks, to urge us to do that extra push-up.

You'll probably come to the realization fairly early in your training that the male students in your school are stronger than you are. In most cases, this will be true. However, don't be intimidated by it. Martial arts training encompasses such a variety of abilities—from flexibility to strength to endurance to intelligence—that where you may not rank in the top of your class in one area, you'll have the opportunity to rank high in other areas. If your male classmates are stronger than you, aim to be more flexible than they are, or aim to have more endurance, or aim to be smarter than they are. However, remember that, as discussed earlier, excelling in the martial arts isn't about ranking in the top of your class in anything; it's about moving at your own pace and achieving your own goals.

When it comes to strength, I'm about average among the women in my class—I won't even compare myself to the men. And since I'm not unusually flexible, I concentrate my efforts instead on endurance, speed, and form.

I've increased my endurance and speed by supplementing my training with jogging and sprinting. When sparring with a large, strong opponent, I'll use my endurance and speed to move around a great deal in an effort to tire him or her out. When an opening occurs, I come in quickly, deliver a technique, then get out before my opponent has a chance to throw a technique. My endurance training also prevents me from getting winded when performing katas.

I've improved my form by concentrating on the details of a move—its timing, its angle, its shape. Because I'm a detail-oriented person to begin with, I don't mind the repetition involved in dissecting the mechanics of every move that makes up a kata. The result is katas that are in many cases cleaner and sharper than other students' katas.

I also came to a point early in my martial arts training when I realized I wouldn't get any stronger. Instead of getting frustrated, I accepted it. Though I probably could have trained harder in class, and supplemented my training with a full weight-lifting program, I didn't. I was satisfied with my level of achievement. After all, I didn't take up a martial art with the specific goal of getting stronger. It was simply a pleasant side effect of my training.

That's why it's important to decide early in your training what you want to achieve from it. Try making a list. It might be numbered from one to five, with one being the most important achievement you have in mind. My list looks something like this:

1. Keep in shape.
2. Expose myself to something new.
3. Spend less time watching television.
4. Meet new people.
5. Work out without having to think about what I'm going to wear.

Others may want to relieve stress or experience the meditational and spiritual benefits of martial arts.

At the end of class, when students are seated on the floor according to rank, my instructor will occasionally ask them to briefly describe why they decided to study a martial art. Though you usually hear the same responses—"for the tough workout," "so I can protect myself"—once in a while you'll hear something original. (Rare is the student who admits he or she took up a martial art to get a black belt, although it's probably the driving force for many students.)

If your instructor doesn't require his students to perform this mental exercise, do it yourself. In addition to your what-I-want-to-achieve list, as you train in a martial art, keep another list—it can even be a mental list—of the benefits of training you didn't expect to obtain. Improved coordination might be on that list, as well as the ability to think more clearly, to make well-thought-out decisions, to sense someone's presence without actually seeing them. My list, which is continually changing, looks something like this:

1. Met the man who would become my husband.
2. Gained the ability to remain calm in a crisis situation.
3. Increased my self-confidence.
4. Improved my posture.
5. Body shape switched from pearlike to T-shaped.

Avoiding Injury

Naturally, no martial arts student expects to get injured. But before you take up a martial art, understand that to an extent it goes with the territory, regardless of your degree of flexibility and strength. On the other hand, most people who take up a sport incur injuries. If you're completely against this fact of sports life, then perhaps you'd be better off working out on your own or at a gym. Then again be prepared to accept the boredom that comes with that form of workout.

When I think back to my early training, I realize that the injuries I incurred were easily preventable. It was often as a result of my own nervousness and trying to impress the instructor and my classmates that I injured myself. It was also as a result of not remaining focused that I incurred injuries.

As a new student, you should constantly remind yourself to focus on yourself and your instructor. Sometimes it's worthwhile to block out the other students when you're not working with them. If students are practicing techniques as a group in front of a mirror, which is a common drill in my school, focus on yourself and how the instructor is performing the moves. If the instructor is walking around the class correcting individual students, focus on the black belts in the class, who are often placed in front of the room for that sole purpose. Don't think about the new student next to you, or the yellow, green, or brown belts in front of you. (Yes, in most martial arts schools, new students are placed in the back of the class during drills. While it's not easy to see yourself in the mirror, it's a lot less stressful than being placed in front of the class. Moreover, a good instructor will make sure that you can see yourself in the mirror and that you receive the instruction you need.)

Sparring probably accounts for about 80 percent of all injuries incurred in the martial arts. Despite the fact that as a new student you'll be watched so closely that the chances of getting injured are minute, it's nevertheless important to keep yourself focused—almost to the point at which you might even disregard who you're sparring with. Think of your opponent as one long tree trunk with branches aimed at you. Consider each branch as it comes your way, blocking it, then throwing a technique to hit the trunk. This way you'll remove yourself from the personal aspect of sparring, and concentrate all your efforts on the technical side, thus decreasing your chances of injury.

Also, don't feel pressured to always listen to your instructor, especially when it comes to sparring. For instance, if you are partnered with someone you don't trust—maybe he hits harder than he should, or his punches seem to have a habit of landing in your chest—don't get too close to your opponent despite the fact that your instructor may be yelling at you to go in and take a shot. Your instructor doesn't want to see you get injured. He simply wants to push you to new limits. But sometimes you're better off following your own instincts.

Generally, fewer injuries are incurred when practicing take-down techniques one-on-one with other students. The pace is often slower, and there's less competition than in sparring. If, however, during these workouts you feel the other student is roughhousing you, tell him or her to take it easy. I recall often screaming internally to myself that my partner must be crazy or else he wouldn't be twisting my wrist so hard, or throwing me to the floor with such force. (I'd even go home mumbling to myself what a jerk the guy was.) Unfortunately, only I could hear my internal screaming. You have to speak up, and a simple reminder to take it easy is usually sufficient.

When working one-on-one with a student, again focus your attention on what you are doing. If you twist your partner's wrist too far, she will indicate for you to stop by tapping or lightly slapping you, herself, or (if she's lying on the ground) the floor. If you perform the technique incorrectly, your partner will correct you. Listen to your partner's advice, but don't be apologetic or embarrassed that you made a mistake. Simply take the advice, focus, and proceed. If neither of you fully understands the move, don't be shy. Simply motion to the instructor or a high-ranking student—usually by raising your hand—that you require assistance.

Most of the injuries you are likely to incur or witness will range from bruises to jammed fingers or toes. Sometimes you'll notice blood on someone's uniform, which is often the result of a scab having been opened or a small cut incurred from a student's fingernail penetrating a partner's skin.

Bruises are another common injury. Karate students routinely incur bruises on their forearms from blocking oncoming punches. I've even jammed fingers by trying to block an oncoming punch. Instead of making a fist with my hand and blocking with my forearm, I left my hand opened and hit my opponent's arm straight on with my middle and ring fingers, causing the joints to be pushed together. Though uncomfortable, most instructors will allow students to train, though not at full capacity, with a jammed finger or toe. (Unfortunately, in my experience, jammed fingers never completely heal, which means you'll never get those favorite rings on them again.)

Most of the more severe injuries you are likely to incur or witness include simple fractures, sprains, and strains. A fracture is a breakage in the bone, ranging from a crack to a smashed bone. (If the bone breaks through the skin, it's called a compound fracture, and at no point in your training should you witness or incur something like this.)

A sprain occurs when a joint is forced beyond its normal range of motion, injuring the ligament, which attaches the bones together. A strain occurs when a muscle, tendon, or group of muscles is overstetched. The best defense against a sprain is to warm up properly prior to class. If an injury does occur, a well-prepared instructor will have on hand packets of ice to apply to the injured area. Generally, students with fractures, sprains, and strains must stop training until some healing takes place. After that the student slowly works her way back into a regular training regimen.

Training Equipment

There's an old photograph that is often reproduced in karate books. The blurry black-and-white image depicts eight martial artists training outdoors with different types of training apparatuses. One item resembles a rock with a stick stuck into it; another looks like a cinder block with a handle carved into it; and yet another consists of a set of large jars—probably filled with sand or pebbles—with raised lips. One man—and they are all men—is wearing what can only be described as platform flip-flops, the base of which is probably made of a heavy, solid material.

Though primitive by today's standards, the training equipment depicted in the photo is to a large extent still popular among martial artists, especially karate students. The rock with the stick stuck into it? That's a "chishi." Updated versions of it are still used to strengthen grips and wrists. Its user simply grabs it, then slowly swings it around in a controlled manner. She might swing it in front of her body or behind her head, using one hand or both hands.

In addition to the chishi, many types of training equipment have been developed to strengthen the all-important grip. But if tradition isn't part of your training curriculum, you may never be introduced to such equipment. To strengthen students' grips, a teacher might instruct his students to perform simple exercises. He might have students strengthen their grips by extending their arms straight out and squeezing their hands closed into a fist and then opened flat—several hundred times. The same can be achieved by gripping tennis balls or small smooth stones.

The gripping jars depicted in the picture, called "nigiri-game" (NIGĒRĒ-GAMĀ), are also designed to strengthen grips. New students would generally start out gripping the raised lips of two empty jars. Later they might add weight to the jars by filling them with sand. Real show-offs might even oil the mouths of the jars to make them slippery.

A traditional karate school might also have a "makiwara" (MAKĒ-WARA), which is basically a striking post. Originally constructed of straw rope wrapped around the top of a wooden board, today's makiwara is often made of black rubber. Karate students strike it to harden the knuckles of their index and middle fingers, which are the first point of contact for a straight punch. Students can also kick the post to harden the sides of their feet.

Today's martial artists are less likely to be found kicking or punching traditional makiwaras, or swinging chishis around their heads. Traditional makiwara posts have been replaced by canvas-covered makiwara boards that can be held by one student while another strikes it. As with traditional makiwaras, it's still relatively easy to break the skin on your knuckles using these boards. Some instructors encourage students to strike boards or pads until their knuckles are raw and bleeding. I always shied away from this. The minute I feel the skin on my knuckles breaking, or see any trace of blood, I ease up on my punches. No amount of praise from my instructor is worth bleeding over.

But not all martial arts emphasize the need for strength like karate. Certainly, tae kwon do and jeet kune emphasize powerful moves. But many styles of martial arts—kung fu, aikido, judo, jujitsu—don't involve such intensive conditioning. Still, you should be familiar with the most common types of training equipment if only to help you choose the style best for you.

More common types of training equipment fall into two categories: pads and bags. Pads are usually made of foam wrapped in vinyl or canvas; bags often come filled with cotton fiber wrapped in vinyl or canvas. Both pads and bags enable students to strike and kick at full force.

Small pads, usually about ten inches by ten inches, are held closely at chest level by means of cloth handles. It's important that the student holding the pad exhales each time her partner strikes it. The problem for female students is obvious. Depending on how big you are on top, taking blows to your chest can range from annoying to painful to embarrassing—to all three. The most logical move an instructor can make is to pair off female students with female students. But unfortunately logic doesn't always prevail in a martial arts school. If your instructor isn't in the habit of taking a woman's anatomy into consideration when pairing up students for this type of exercise, tell your male partner straight out to take it easy.

Large pads, which are about two feet long and a foot and a half wide, are held in front of the body also by means of cloth handles. Because of their size, these pads enable students to throw a greater variety of strikes and kicks. They also offer students holding them more protection than their smaller counterparts. Manufacturers have recently come out with large pads containing air and foam, which together absorb more impact than pads containing only foam. If your school has these, consider it fairly progressive. On the other hand, schools with the most-advanced equipment pay for it with students' tuition dollars, and may have to subsequently charge high tuition fees.

Pads that are worn on the forearms are frequently used in martial arts styles that utilize kicks, such as karate and tae kwon do. Like with the other pads, the wearer simply slips her forearms into the cloth handles on the back of the pads. Unlike other pads, these are probably the most comfortable pads for women to wear. Instead of holding them in one place, such as the chest area, a student can raise her arms high, prompting her partner to extend her leg high to strike what might be an opponent's head. Or she can lower her arm, prompting her partner to execute what would be a kick to an imaginary opponent's leg.

I've always preferred punching bags to pads for the simple and obvious reason that I don't have to hold them. (Although, to keep them in place, the bags may have to be held if a particularly strong student is kicking or punching them.) Punching or striking bags hang from the ceiling or are attached by two elastic ropes—one that extends to the ceiling, the other to the floor. Punching bags are also the one type of training equipment you're likely to encounter that most resembles a person. By imagining that the bag is your boss, enemy, or the customer service representative who never heard of the words "thank you," you can punch and kick your aggressions away.

Until you've stepped up to a small hanging punching bag—the kind you often see boxers using—you'll never realize how difficult it is to work with. Here coordination is the name of the game. Not only must you hit it, but you've also got to develop timing and speed. It takes a lot of practice, which is something many students, especially women, avoid, because to become proficient at it, you've got to be willing to look like an uncoordinated fool. After your first few tries, you'll wonder how you manage to walk and chew gum at the same time. But keep at it. You'll increase your upper body strength and size, develop a superior sense of timing and speed, and impress the hell out of every male student in your class.

Large hanging punching bags are a lot easier to practice with. Their size makes them easy to strike at and actually hit. But they're also solid, so be careful. A weak punch thrown at it could result in an injury to the fingers or the wrist. Hard kicks to it could result in bruises or dark red marks. Despite the fact that manufacturers have come out with hanging bags that contain water instead of cotton fiber, and therefore allow students to perform high-impact workouts without incurring injuries, I've yet to see one of these devices in a school.

The best advice is to start out easy. Throw some soft punches, then work your way up until you're throwing hard strikes and kicks, but aren't uncomfortable doing so. No matter how loud or forceful your instructor yells for you to "go harder," listen to your inner voice. After all, it's you who will go home with bruises, not him.

In addition to striking and kicking pads, and wearing them when sparring, martial arts students, especially judoists, also roll on padded mats. Some schools have wall-to-wall padding on all the floors; others cover one side of the training floor with padding, the other with a hard wood spring floor; still others bring the mats out on an as-needed basis, then store them when not in use. Either way, they will be your best friend when starting out in your chosen martial art. Just knowing that there's two inches of dense foam awaiting you as you take your first few rolls or falls is enough of an assurance to let you concentrate on what you're doing rather than whether it will hurt.

In addition to pads and bags, you may also train with such equipment as medicine balls and padded mitts. Padded mitts used in the martial arts resemble stiff baseball gloves. They fit over your hands and are used with a partner to improve aim, focus, and timing. The student wearing the mitts moves her hands around, creating a moving target for her opponent to strike at.

In my school, medicine balls are passed around, several at a time, while the class stands in a circle. The idea is to throw it into your neighbor's gut as hard as you can. The problem is sometimes your neighbor aims too high or too low. A word of advice here is to try to stand next to women or students who have good aim and don't throw so hard, or, at the very least, students who are your size. If the person standing next to you is a foot or so taller than you, he might inadvertently throw the ball into your chest. Ideally, the ball should hit you in your stomach area. Always exhale when the ball hits your midsection, and understand that it's okay to tell your neighbor to throw the ball softer.

While one could argue the merits of throwing a heavy ball into someone's gut, it seems to me that some martial arts enthusiasts went a bit too far when they developed a piece of equipment known as the leg-stretching machine. Resembling a seat with wings, these machines hold one occupant, who fits her legs into the "wings," then adjusts them until her legs form a 180-degree angle. Personally, it seems more suited for a torture chamber than a martial arts school. If you can't do this naturally, I don't think your body should be forced into this position.

And, finally, for the martial artist who dreams of glory days where she's breaking boards before crowds of hundreds of cheering fans, there's the rebreakable board. Made of plastic, the rebreakable board can be broken, put easily back together, and rebroken hundreds of times. Hitting the board is supposed to be like striking a three-quarter inch piece of pine—not exactly the kind of activity most of us look for when taking up a martial art.

8. Life Imitates the Martial Arts

"Women are just starting to get the recognition they deserve. I'd rather train females any day than males. They don't have the egos and the attitudes. If females see somebody that's tougher and stronger, it makes them work harder."

—Male karate school owner and instructor, as quoted in the *New York Times*, November, 7, 1993

Do WOMEN IN the martial arts really try harder than their male counterparts? Many women in the martial arts seem to think so. Some have described feeling pressure to prove themselves more proficient than the men in their schools. Maybe women just try harder. Or perhaps women martial artists try to be accommodating in order to avoid "rocking the boat" or drawing attention to themselves.

Much of this probably stems from being the sole female, or one of a small group of females, in a martial arts school dominated by men. Certainly, in any setting in which you represent a minority, there is always the pressure to prove yourself, or at least not to make yourself stand out. It's not unlike women's relatively recent mass migration into the work force. In the '70s, women were relegated to secretarial jobs, and the gender issue loomed large over their heads. Not until more women started making inroads into management did their male counterparts focus less on gender. Likewise, not until the first pioneering women martial artists began moving up the ranks did male martial artists view them as capable opponents rather than simply women.

That women have made significant inroads in the business world only in the past few decades isn't the only similarity shared by women in the martial arts and business. Both the martial arts and business require similar skills. To excel at both, you need to develop the ability to strategize, work one-on-one with different types of partners, and learn when to ask for help and how to give it. And as much as the martial arts require inner reflection, the sport also demands that practitioners work well on a team level—concepts that have worked well for Japanese businesses.

Even the philosophical teachings inherent in the martial arts have been adopted in the business world. For example, strategies of ancient Japanese philosophers have found a home in the business sections of bookstores. In his book, *The Japanese Art of War*, author Thomas Cleary describes the martial arts principles that to this day are commonly found in Japanese corporate boardrooms. The martial arts philosophy of learning every aspect of the sport, no matter how simple or intricate, he says, has been "applied by the Japanese in the corporate world of the latter half of the twentieth century, and is one of the major factors supporting well-known technical and sociological successes seen in Japanese business and industry."

Many of us have also witnessed examples of Japanese businessmen being yelled at to the point of tears by militant-like teachers. Cleary traces this style of training, used in Japanese personnel development, to the "hard" martial arts that stress force and strength to overcome an opponent. On a lighter note, the author links the ability to use the mind to solve problems with the spiritual tradition of Zen, which, he says, is generally found in the "soft" martial arts. To overcome their opponents, practitioners of Zen rely on knowledge, he says, or what is called the "art of the advantage" as opposed to force, or the "art of the sword." In the United States, martial arts practitioners who sell for a living have noted that their studies have enhanced their ability to understand and respond to their prospects, and given them psychological insights into their competitors and clients.

Opening Doors to Women

As explained in a previous chapter, most martial arts instructors are small-business people. They are entrepreneurial and, hopefully, driven as much by the profit motive as by the desire to attract and train the best students. But to succeed in both endeavors, many martial arts instructors discovered long ago that they had to open their schools to both male and female students in order to survive in this competitive business environment.

The influx of women into the martial arts has infused schools with more personalities and opinions than ever before. Consequently, there is more room for personality clashes and differences of opinion. Just as in the workplace, men have had to adjust to the presence of women in martial arts schools. But in the workplace, the only interaction with other people is on a verbal level. Anything beyond that might be construed as sexual harassment.

In martial arts schools, verbal and physical interaction are mandatory. While talking during class is generally prohibited, working one-on-one with a student does require some discussion involving how to stand, which hand to use and when, and how to correct a move. And, obviously, it involves a great deal of physical interaction. It's no wonder, then, that opening martial arts doors to women has been a rude awakening to some male students, many of whom have been forced to interact with females on levels unfamiliar and uncomfortable to them.

Actually, when you think about it, male martial artists are asked for a lot. They are asked to grab, grapple, and strike at female students—no simple task given the many high-profile sexual harassment cases we've seen in the past few years. Chances are good that during your martial arts training, you will hear female students complain that so-and-so intentionally hit her in the chest or focused his eyes solely on her chest area as they sparred. Sometimes it's enough to make male students avoid having to work with female students. What you end up with is a situation where male students avoid female students—and even female students avoid male students.

Watch this pressure come to life when your teacher instructs students to pair up with a partner in order to practice one-on-one takedowns. What commonly happens during the next couple of frenzied minutes is male students seek out their male counterparts, and females seek out their female counterparts. After the dust settles, all the students will be standing beside a partner, except for two students—one male, the other female—each looking around in hopes of finding a similar-sex student hiding in the corner. When they realize there are no other students, they clumsily approach each other.

Don't let this kind of situation deter you from entering the martial arts. The above example is a worse-case scenario. It usually happens to a much lesser extent. What's more, there are things you can do to reduce the tension that may arise when you are working with a male student who is uncomfortable working with a female student. Start by trying to set an example in the school. Dismiss the thought that it matters who you work with. You shouldn't care if you are that last student standing without a partner while a male student pretends not to see you. Make eye contact with that student, go over, and nonchalantly stand by him.

MARTIAL MAXIM: AS YOU BECOME ACCUSTOMED TO WORKING WITH EVERY STUDENT IN YOUR SCHOOL, YOU'LL FIND YOU'RE LESS INHIBITED INTERACTING WITH PEOPLE OUTSIDE YOUR SCHOOL AS WELL.

To overcome the tension with your partner, clear your mind and focus on the task at hand. Nervousness will only lead to mistakes and perhaps even injuries. So concentrate your thoughts on what you're doing, not who you're doing it with. That alone should put your partner at ease and allow the two of you to focus on the moves the class as a whole is practicing.

If the issue continues to play a major part in the school, talk to your instructor. But before you make any suggestions, buffer what you're about to say (and this applies to almost any time you make suggestions to your instructor) with something to the effect of "I just wanted to bring to your attention something you may not be aware of." This will give your instructor an out by allowing him to say something like, "I'm aware of it, but maybe you should fill me in on the details."

You might suggest to the instructor that he personally pair off students in order to encourage greater interaction. He might also take the time during a class to explain why it is necessary to work with students of different sizes and sexes. Not only will you be called on to demonstrate moves with different partners during a promotional test, but should you ever be attacked outside your school, you will be better prepared to protect yourself. Women, particularly, should make it a point to work with all the male students in their classes in order to get a feel for how their moves work with attackers of various sizes. What's it like to be grabbed from behind by a six-foot man versus a five-foot man? Working with the largest number of students possible will let you find out.

Of course, some people are simply uncomfortable working with anyone they don't know—male or female. To these individuals, the mere thought of practicing a martial art with a stranger turns them off. To get around these fears, many people will join with a friend, significant other, or spouse.

These people often join a school together in the belief that they'll encourage and push each other to study a martial art, and to an extent, it is true. On the one hand, it's beneficial in that it encourages two people to join when individually they never would. But it can also lead to two students completely dependent on each other. When it's time to pick a partner, these students often turn toward each other, and since they're joining at the same level, they're usually standing right next to each other, making it easy for them to work solely together. In more severe cases, one friend will decide to quit, and the other friend will just follow.

If you join with a partner, do not let yourself be overly influenced by his or her comments and criticisms. Hopefully, you joined the school because it met all of your criteria. Always evaluate the school and the teacher according to your own standards. If you like the school, the style, and the teacher as much as your partner does, you'll be fortunate because you'll have a companion to encourage you to attend class and to practice with you when you are not in class.

Setting Standards

Besides making some male students nervous, another result of martial arts schools opening their doors to women is that it has put a spotlight on school standards. Some claim it has diminished standards—that in order to draw and keep female students, schools have had to make the workouts and the promotional tests easier. However, such a theory doesn't hold water. If a school really did this, it would lose its male students too. What's more, today's female athletes are no lightweights—most are every bit the athletes as the men, and some a good deal more.

Of course, there are schools that have low standards. However, the standards apply to all the students. Often, you will find students in these schools who are more interested in getting a black belt than in learning an art with any lasting value. Again, it is up to you to decide if a school meets your standards. And since there are no set industry standards, it is up to each student to assess whether a school meets her own. On the other hand, there are those who say female students have raised school standards. With more students entering schools, these people claim, instructors can be pickier, encouraging good students to excel and inferior students or troublemakers to leave.

MARTIAL MAXIM: STANDARDS VARY FROM SCHOOL TO SCHOOL. ACCORDING TO ONE SEVENTH-DEGREE BLACK BELT WHO RUNS A KARATE SCHOOL IN NEW YORK CITY, NEW SCHOOLS TEND TO GIVE A MORE MILD WORKOUT SO NO ONE QUITS. "IT'S COMMERCIALISM VERSUS TRADITIONALISM," HE SAYS.

That's why it pays to choose your school well, taking the time to evaluate the style, the teacher, and students. Remember, you could spend up to four or five hours a week there for as many as five or more years. Changing schools may dampen your enthusiasm as you try to adopt to a new teacher, teaching style, and students, hoping all the while that the school will be better than the last one. If you take the time to properly evaluate a school, you will find yourself surrounded by a dynamic group of people, male and female, for years to come. It will be an atmosphere in which students are more concerned with learning and helping out their fellow classmates than with trying to prove that they're stronger, tougher, and smarter than anyone else in the class.

Teachers Make the Adjustment, Too

Students are not the only ones who have had to adjust to a more diverse martial arts. As more women enter the martial arts, teachers have had to develop new management and communications skills. Should female students be pushed as hard as male students? If they request it, should female students be exempt from having to spar with certain male students? Is it okay to keep a female student after class to go over some forms, or might that be misconstrued among the other students? If the men have showers available to them, should showers be installed for the women? Even though there are generally more male students than female students, should the women's dressing room be the same size as the men's dressing room? Instructors who do not have the luxury of building a new school or remodeling an old one must make hard decisions that could eventually benefit one group of students at the expense of another.

If your instructor grapples with decisions such as these, consider yourself lucky. At least the teacher is sensitive to these issues. Though few and far between, it is not unheard of for instructors to take advantage of their female students. Martial arts magazines have chronicled instances of instructors more interested in going out with a female student than in teaching her a martial art. In one such article, a woman described her breakup with her instructor, whom she had been dating. She continued to study with him, but found her sparring sessions with him became more and more abusive, with the instructor at one point punching her in the face, then claiming she walked into it.

You may never encounter occurrences like these inside martial arts schools. But it does pay to remember that instructors are only human. They are not to be worshiped, but rather respected—and that respect should be returned. Most students who have found themselves in negative situations

174 IN THE DOJO

with their instructors probably saw the warning signs in advance. If you sense something is wrong, chances are there is.

Most martial arts instructors live by an above-average code of conduct. Most make themselves responsible for weeding out negative students. They maintain a balance between the gender of their students, as well as their ages and belt levels. Most wouldn't want a school full of brown and black belts, and most wouldn't dwell on one group at the expense of another. When an instructor wants to focus on the black belts in his school, or on only students with, say, a green belt or higher, he schedules special classes accordingly. He does not dwell on high-ranking students in a class that also contains white and yellow belts. Likewise, most instructors would not want mostly male students in his class—such a mix would discourage females from joining. In fact, some instructors favor their top female students because these students act as a powerful draw to prospective female students. In addition to keeping martial arts schools prosperous by drawing the best and the brightest, such a healthy attitude encourages diversity, which makes for a more interesting school.

Fighting Egos

If you choose your school well, you may not find any tension among the male and female students there. But chances are you will find egos. It has been said that Hollywood's portrayal of martial artists as possessing superhuman strength and uncanny intuition has attracted to the martial arts individuals of both genders who have low self-esteem and large egos. These are the kinds of students who believe that after just a few lessons they are ready to take on the world. You would think that a couple of ill-timed blocks on these students' parts would keep their egos from inflating. But that's rarely the case.

Chances are good that there will be at least one student in your class with an ego. This student may be louder than the others and more critical in an unconstructive way, and may consistently put down other students (especially when those "other" students aren't within earshot). From experience, I can tell you that they aren't, as you would expect, outstanding students. In fact, they are usually just mediocre. The big ego isn't there as a result of being especially blessed athletically; on the contrary, the ego is usually there as a shield, protecting its owner from admitting his or her inadequacies.

I've seen everything from students who spend more time staring at their hair in the mirrors that line the inside wall of a school than at their forms, to students who turn up their noses at low-ranking students, to students who strut their stuff around the floor as though they were somehow a cut above the mere mortals with whom they share the dojo. How do you deal with these students? They can't be ignored, because eventually you'll have to work with them. In my experience, I've found that treating them no differently from other students probably drives them crazier than if you were to confront them or try to ignore them.

If your teacher carries the biggest ego in the school, you've got a problem. Hopefully, however, you decided not to join that school. But there are several things inherent in martial arts schools that prevent egos from spinning out of control: the adherence to traditional values and to etiquette and manners. Requiring students to address one another politely, bow and thank one another goes a long way in keeping them humble. (Certainly, the erosion of manners in today's society is one reason so many parents send their children to martial arts schools.)

Pass the Etiquette, Please

Probably more time is spent on maintaining a high level of etiquette in the martial arts than in any other sport. Certainly, martial artists are expected to go beyond a mere handshake, which is probably the most common, and in some sports only, means of showing good sportsmanship. Though the degree of etiquette varies from school to school, I've not seen any school that doesn't expect its students to show respect for their peers and the teacher by bowing to, thanking, acknowledging, and encouraging fellow students.

This type of formalized behavior acts as a balancing agent against the inherent aggressive nature of the sport. It's difficult to remain angry at someone who accidentally hits you after he gives you a sincere handshake following the match. And by formally reaching out your hand to your opponent before a sparring match, you're introducing the human element into what is taught to be an nonemotional exercise. (During your training, you'll be sure to hear your instructor telling you numerous times to wear an expressionless face as you spar—whether you take a hit or you throw a perfect one into your opponent.)

Bowing is probably the most-used gesture of respect in the martial arts. For example, it signals the beginning or end of something. Students bow before a sparring match, then afterward. Bowing is also commonly done before and after stepping onto the training floor, and performing prearranged forms and one-on-one practice drills.

Bowing is also done when greeting other students, and not just high-ranking ones. Some schools may only require that students bow before high-ranking students, but it doesn't hurt to get into the habit of bowing before all students. In fact, once you enter the school, the formalities typically start. A scenario might go like this: You enter the school and bow toward the floor before entering the dressing room. (You would also take off your shoes prior to entering the dressing room if you have to walk on the training floor to get to the room.) If you pass students along the way, you're likely to have to bow to them and greet them with a traditional "Oss," which is a common greeting used in some martial schools and is the English equivalent of saying hello. Once in the dressing room, it is fairly informal—probably the most informal room in the school. Still, it doesn't hurt to greet everyone there with an "Oss" minus the bow.

MARTIAL MAXIM: BOWING DEPICTS MUTUAL RESPECT, SO THE SAME AMOUNT OF SERIOUSNESS SHOULD BE PUT INTO EACH BOW, WHETHER IT BE TO YOUR TEACHER, A SEASONED STUDENT, OR A NEW STUDENT.

Once you leave the dressing room, you'll bow before stepping onto the training floor. Then, again, you'll greet fellow students with a bow and an "Oss"—and perhaps even a handshake. Most schools limit conversation to short familiarities, followed by talk related to the martial arts: "Can you help me with my kata?" "I was practicing my blocks, and was having trouble keeping my wrist straight. Can we work on it together?" and so forth.

Whether you work with a partner or decide to work on some moves solo prior to class, take a moment to assess where you will sit when the teacher instructs students to line up. This will make it easier to find your place. In many schools, it is actually more difficult for the low-ranking belts to determine where they will fall in line because they often fall at the back of the line. What's more, all students are expected to line up quickly. In my school, black belts sit up front with the instructor, facing the rest of the students. The highest brown belt takes her place at the front of a line facing the instructor and black belts, with the next highest-ranking student standing to her right, and so on until four or five students fill the first line. Then the next highest-ranking student starts a second line by taking her place behind the highest-ranking brown belt, and so on until the lowest ranking student falls into line in the back.

If you were a white belt trying to figure out where you fall into line, you would in this case count the number of higher-ranking belts, keeping in mind any students still in the dressing room who might make it out in time to line up, then determine the number of white belts who joined the school before you, as they are considered more advanced than you. Now you have the number of students who line up before you. You can also simply locate the student who precedes you in rank, wait until he or she lines up, then fall into place behind him or her—but then you are relying on that student's ability to figure out your place in line.

Once the instructor walks onto the floor, students stop whatever it is they are doing, then upon his command, they line up according to rank, standing rigid with arms shooting straight down at their sides, hands clenched in a fist. The instructor then stands at the head of the class, sometimes with the black belts, depending on the school. He indicates for the class to bow, then sit on the floor. Once seated, students are instructed by the teacher to meditate for a minute or two, followed by a bow from the seated position. Then students stand and begin their warm-up exercises.

As explained before, during class, you'll bow several times, before and after one-on-one takedown drills, katas, and sparring matches. When class ends, you'll sit according to rank once again, and meditate and bow. You'll also bow before leaving the floor, and then perhaps as you leave the school.

Just entering and leaving the school, and passing, say, two students each way, you'll bow six times. Say during the class you perform five katas, spar three times, and practice four takedown drills, you'll bow another twenty-four times. That's a total of thirty bows per class! Therefore, it pays to know how to do it correctly.

Bowing looks simple, until you try it for the first time. Most new students make the same mistakes: staring at the floor as they bend down, bowing too quickly, pushing their shoulders upward, and slapping their arms against their sides before bowing as though they are in the army, not the dojo, and a sergeant is asking them to snap to attention.

To bow from a standing position, place your feet together at the heels with the toes pointing outward at about a fifteen-degree angle. Standing straight with the chin tucked in, mouth lightly closed, shoulders lowered, arms at the sides with the hands open, thumbs tucked in, and palms resting on the thighs, bend at the waist at a fifteen-degree angle, keeping a straight line from the head to the hips. Pause for a couple of seconds before raising yourself back to the original straight standing position. All of this should be performed in one breath.

Bowing from a sitting position is similar to that of a standing position. Students are generally required to bow from a seated position at the beginning and end of class, as well as during class when students work one-on-one from a seated position, practicing wrist grabs and other moves that concentrate solely on hand technique. Bowing from a seated position is basically the same as from a standing position. From a formal seated position—sitting on the backs of your shins—with the palms of the hands resting lightly on the thighs, slide down the hands to the floor, with the hands pointed slightly inward and the tips of the index fingers slightly apart. Lean forward as the hands and forearms touch the floor lightly. While bowing, keep your backside seated. After bowing, return to the upright formal seated position, returning your hands to their original position and looking straight in front of you.

One thing to remember about bowing: It signals respect, not gullibility. As you lean forward at the waist from a standing position, don't take your eyes off your opponent. Your opponent probably won't take a swing at you while you're bowing, but at one time in the history of the sport, it was not unheard of. Also, do not let the quiet, slow pace of a bow put you off guard. I've seen students use bowing to their advantage. Just before a sparring match, as both students rise slowly from their bows, then get in the ready positions, one student will quickly pounce on her opponent the instant the instructor gives the command to begin sparring. Nine times out of ten, the other student, still at ease from bowing, will be taken completely by surprise, and lose the point.

Another advantageous way to use a bow is while performing it. A powerful look thrown as you bend down and find yourself face to face with your opponent can be almost as offsetting as a strong punch. Just compare the difference in eye contact between a new student and a high-ranking student. New students bowing before their partners often wear a frightened, submissive look. You can almost hear them thinking, "Please don't hurt me." High-ranking students generally keep their eyebrows steady and chin tucked in, and look straight into their opponent's eyes, wearing a serious, I-mean-business expression.

Don't be like a lot of students who eventually consider bowing unnecessary—like drivers who don't bother signaling a lane change. As with all martial arts etiquette, bowing maintains tradition and discipline. Bowing also acts as a balancing agent, offsetting the aggressive nature of the sport with civilized behavior.

There are times, however, when etiquette takes a backseat to more important matters. It's okay to step off the floor without bowing if you feel you're going to get sick. It's also all right to stop sparring in the middle of a match if you get injured and feel you'll only worsen the injury if you continue.

I remember the first time I had the air knocked out of me during a sparring match. I lay on the floor in disbelief that I had been hit and that it was so difficult to catch my breath. I certainly wasn't worrying about finishing the match, and neither was my instructor.

9. Three Typical Training Sessions

NOW THAT YOU HAVE BEEN introduced to the basics of martial arts training, you should feel prepared to confidently begin your search for the right style and school for you. You may already be anticipating the first time you walk into a martial arts school. Will there be other students there observing the class? Will the instructor come over and speak with me? What will be the ratio of men to women? Will there be a place for me to sit and observe a class?

But walking into a martial arts school for the first time is just one of many firsts you'll experience. There's the first time a student lunges toward an opponent with the perfect amount of grace and power. There's the first time a student summons up the courage to shout out a full-fledged abdominal shout, surprising herself more than the students around her. There's the first time a student realizes the power she can bring to her punch just by throwing her hip into it.

And, for new students in most martial arts styles, there are the really big firsts: the first test, the first class, and the first sparring session. The following hypothetical scenarios are designed to help you experience these three special firsts.

The First Class

Tricia didn't walk into aikido blind. She did a lot of research and was able to rule out other styles. Judo was too competitive for her, and involved too much grabbing and pulling. Tae kwon do and its high-flying kicks didn't suit her either. And karate placed too much emphasis on strength. Now aikido, with its emphasis on the mind—relaxing it, focusing it, and centering it—that appealed to her.

So why was she so nervous walking into the aikido school to take her first class? She had been to the school before, observed a couple of classes, and spoke at length with the head instructor, who struck her as an understanding, intelligent individual.

As she entered the school, Tricia noticed that everything looked the same as it did last time she was there. Mats covered the floor as some students moved back and forth over them practicing breathing exercises designed to develop their chi. Other students worked their wrists. Still others practiced rolls, placing their hands out in front of them, rolling along their arms, across their backs, then landing on their feet as though throwing the human body to the ground was the most natural thing a person could do.

The students were all wearing karate-like uniforms; Tricia wore sweatpants and a T-shirt. Since this was her first class, Tricia was allowed to wear this attire. After her third class, however, she would have to wear a uniform if she wanted to continue training.

After a few minutes, the teacher steps onto the floor and walks to the front of the class. He wastes no time instructing students to line up according to rank and bow toward him. Then general warm-ups are performed, including one unique to aikido: knee walking. Students kneel, hands resting flat on the floor with their fingers pointing toward the front of their thighs. Then they lift one knee and plant their foot on the floor, continuing this as they make their way across the training floor. As students perform this exercise, the instructor explains that knee walking indicates respect and shows that you have no intention of taking up an attacking standing posture.

After warm-ups, the instructor describes the techniques that will be practiced during class—forward and backward tumbles, side strikes, shoulder grabs, and wrist locks with throws. Then students pair off, with Tricia instructed to work with a senior student.

As Tricia's partner explains what they will be practicing, she can't help but be drawn to the activity around her. Students grab other students' wrists and almost effortlessly bring their partners to the floor. The motion is smooth, graceful, and surprisingly natural, she thinks, wondering, How long will it be before I can do that?

But before she can contemplate further her future in aikido, Tricia's partner says to her, "Tonight we'll practice breakfalls." After a brief explanation of the basics of breakfalling, Tricia gives it a shot. She crouches on the floor with her arms bent and crossed in front of her at her forearms. At the command from her partner, she falls backward, chin tucked in, and arms unfolding, ending with a slap of her hands on the mat. Then she tries breakfalls from each side, slapping out with just one hand and using the other to protect her face.

After performing what feels like endless numbers of breakfalls, Tricia can feel her hands slightly stinging from hitting the mat and is relieved when her partner says, "That's enough for tonight." That feeling quickly dissipates, however, when she realizes he meant that was enough breakfalls; it was on to the next technique.

Sensing her exasperation at having practiced so many falls, Tricia's partner explains that they will now spend their time standing. Before a proper throw can be executed, he says, you've got to learn the basics of grabbing and stepping. With that, he asks Tricia to stand in front of him and grab his right wrist with her right hand and lead him to her left in a curve, then continue in ever-decreasing circles until a centrifugal force develops. Unsure and slightly nervous, Tricia clumsily grabs his arm. After several adjustments by her partner, she steps forward, then begins her circle, slowly then a little faster until she's in control and he is moving with the force that's developed.

"Now let me try it on you," he says. He grabs her arm and proceeds to start her in a circle. Then without warning, applies a twist of the wrist, and Tricia feels her feet lift off the floor as she softly falls to the mat. "I think I've just been thrown for the first time," she says.

Excited that she is actually practicing aikido, Tricia is ready for more. Unfortunately, an hour has already passed, and end-of-class warm-ups are scheduled to begin in just a few minutes. But before they do, the teacher instructs all students to sit against the wall and observe the five black belts in class as they practice "free play."

With that the most senior black belt stands ready as the second highest-ranking black belt moves in. After successfully throwing the attacker, another black belt takes a shot, and on and on until the fourth black belt attacks. Then the second highest-ranking student takes on the role of defender.

As Tricia watched the black belts toss each other almost effortlessly to the ground, she thought about the last hour and how it had been better than she had anticipated. What was even better, she thought, was that her next class was only a day away.

The First Sparring Session

Michele had observed it many times before. The instant the tae kwon do instructor put forth those four words, "Put on your equipment," a mood filled the air bordering on excitement and trepidation. But as the students put on their head and foot gear, padded gloves, and shin guards, and inserted their plastic mouthpieces, the trepidation subsided and the excitement turned to focused strategizing.

Up until now, Michele had been sparring under the watchful eye of her instructor and various black belts. The pace was slow and no contact was allowed. This exercise allowed her to match the right blocks to certain strikes, and to develop combinations. When one of the black belts she sparred with would throw a straight punch, for example, she would counter with a middle block, followed by a punch to his head and perhaps even a kick to his midsection.

But now, as the class sat in a formal seated position alongside the wall, she somehow knew that today she would spar without the safety net she had become used to. Her instructor had told her she was ready to start sparring like the rest of the advanced yellow belts. That meant picking up considerably the pace to which she had grown accustomed; throwing, and being willing to take, harder punches and kicks; and going one-on-one with the green and brown belts, who tended to be somewhat more aggressive and certainly more careless, than the black belts.

The teacher eyes the line the students have formed along the wall, from the black belts at one end to the white belts at the other end, with brown, green, yellow belts in between. He looks at the brown belts and says, "Mr. Williams."

Within seconds, Mr. Williams is standing perfectly still in the center of the floor, eyes staring straight ahead. "Ms. MacMaster," says the instructor. Instantly, Michele finds herself jumping to her feet and running to take her place in front of Mr. Williams, arms jutting down at her sides, ending in clenched fists. She looks straight at her opponent. He looks confident, skilled, even angry. "At me?" Michele thinks. Then she remembers that half the battle in sparring is maintaining concentration. Michele takes a deep breath and clears her mind of everything except the task at hand.

The instructor shouts the command to bow. With their hands at their sides and their legs together, they bow, neither one of them taking their eyes off each other. Another command echoes from the instructor, and they assume a fighting stance—fists at the ready and one leg back, positioned to kick or sidestep away from a kick. As they step back, they both project deep abdominal shouts.

A third command, and they begin sparring. Michele's opponent wastes no time, lunging into her with a straight punch, which she successfully sidesteps, but a sudden round-house kick plants itself in her midsection, not quite knocking the wind out of her but startling her nonetheless.

The teacher calls for both students to stop. "Are you all right?" he asks Michele, who nods in the affirmative. At this point, Michele's level of determination shoots up several notches.

After a quick admonishment from the instructor, Mr. Williams agrees not to kick or strike with full force—a real no-no in class sparring. "Nothing more than a tap," says the teacher. "Save that other stuff for competition," he adds, referring to point sparring in which martial artists compete for trophies and ribbons.

Both students square off again. This time Mr. Williams doesn't rush in. Michele twitches as if to throw a punch. He falls for the fake, and sidesteps what he interprets as an advance. Then Michele throws a side kick that taps him firmly between his rib cage and hip.

With sweat dripping down her face, Michele feels a rush of excitement. "So that's what it feels like to score a point in sparring," she thinks to herself. Then her attention turns quickly back to Mr. Williams, who, she thinks, is probably annoyed and slightly embarrassed that he was hit by a yellow belt. But with true martial arts spirit, he hardly shows it.

As they resume sparring, Mr. Williams releases a hook punch from the left to the side of Michele's head. With her hands already correctly positioned near her face, she easily blocks it. Then he throws a left jab, which she barely blocks in time.

Now it's her turn again. And since she's only inches from him, Michele strikes with her knee, which causes Mr. Williams to step back.

Using the space she has created between them, as well as her five-foot-seven-inch frame, to her advantage, Michele throws her right leg in a long roundhouse kick at Mr. Williams's head. Predictably, he shifts his head away from the kick, which puts it in direct contact with the back of her right fist, which she has since thrown to the other side of his head.

The instructor yells for both students to stop. They return to the center of the floor, hands at their sides, legs together, heels touching, and bow to each other.

They shake hands, and thank each other. Then they turn and run to their respective places against the wall. Michele glances at the clock and notices that the whole sparring session took no more than about four minutes. She feels the sweat dripping down her back, her hands are shaking slightly, but she feels a sense of accomplishment she has never felt before.

The First Test

Today's class starts like many have over the past five months since Ann started studying karate: Fifteen minutes of warm-ups, followed by practice drills consisting of punches, blocks, and kicks performed in front of the mirrors that line one side of the training floor.

But something was different. The instructor was spending more time than usual on Ann. As he walked the floor correcting students' aim and form, he would stop in front of Ann as she threw straight punches. Then he would place the palm of his hand in front of her punch so he could feel the impact of it. After each punch, he would repeat, "Harder, harder." Then he would tell the class to execute middle blocks to his count. At the count of one—yelled out in the traditional Japanese word, "ichi"—the class would throw the block with their right hands. At the count of two—"ni," in Japanese—every student in the class would throw a left-handed block. Still standing in front of Ann, the instructor would throw a punch at her as she blocked it. "Harder," he would say, adding, "and don't bend your wrist."

It was almost too much for her. If he doesn't stop picking on me, I'll scream, Ann thought. Maybe he sensed her frustration, and stepped to the student besides Ann, stopping to test the strength of his block.

After about fifteen minutes of these drills, Ann was feeling strong but fatigued. She was relieved when the instructor stopped the drills and let students cool down by rotating their hips and shaking out their arms. She was even more relieved when he instructed students to collect their fighting gear and sit against the wall according to rank. That could only mean one thing: the class was about to spar.

Sparring was still new enough to Ann that the instructor wasn't yet allowing her to go at it full force. When the pairs of students would take turns sparring in the middle of the floor, a senior student would sit next to Ann, at the instructor's request, and explain what the two sparring students were doing in the center of the floor. Or, as was the case recently, Ann would spar in slow motion with a senior student, usually Bruce Connor, who went to great lengths to go easy on her.

Expecting the instructor to start by calling the two most

senior students to the middle of the floor, she was caught by surprise when he said, "Miss Turner and Mr. Connor." Bruce was quick to jump up and run to the center of the floor, standing rigid with tight fists and staring straight ahead. It took Ann a few seconds longer to realize she was supposed to do the same. Then it hit her—she was being tested.

Panic, fear, anxiety, stress, and confusion consumed her as she fell into position facing her partner. "Rei" (pronounced RĀY), the instructor said, and the two students bowed to each other. Then the instructor issued the command to begin, and Ann and Bruce set up in a ready position—fists near their faces and right legs back.

Bruce threw the same straight punch he had thrown many times at her during their practice sessions. But Ann's nervousness got the best of her, and instead of blocking it, she walked into it. "Keep going," said the instructor. This time Ann took the lead and threw a roundhouse kick to Bruce's midsection. He blocked it, then threw a controlled punch that stopped just an inch from Ann's face. "Yame," shouted the instructor, and the match ended.

While the instructor continued to call up pairs of students to spar, Ann gathered her composure. She knew her instructor wouldn't test her if he didn't feel she was ready. Besides, if she failed miserably, it would be a direct reflection on him and his teaching abilities. Not wanting to embarrass her teacher, or herself for that matter, Ann became determined to give the test her all.

When the instructor called on her to spar a second time, she sparred better. And when the instructor had her stand in the center of the floor in a low sumo stance that made her legs ache and knees shake, she not only held the position firmly, but she knew the English equivalent of every Japanese term the instructor threw at her. And when the instructor commanded her to perform her kata, she did so flawlessly.

Toward the end of class, as students sat in traditional

formal positions according to rank, Ann was called to the front of the room. Having watched several tests since she started studying karate, Ann knew enough to sit in front of the instructor. He lifted the end of her white belt and wrapped yellow tape around it, then did the same with the other end. She was now a white belt with a yellow tab. Teacher and student bowed to each other, then Ann turned and bowed to the rest of the class. Then she rose and returned to her seated position at the back of the room, amazed at how confident and strong she felt.

10. In the Spirit of Things

MUCH HAS BEEN WRITTEN about the physical and spiritual aspects of the martial arts. Certainly, the physical part is straightforward. Anyone who has taken even one martial arts class will attest that it gave her a strenuous workout—for some, the workout of a lifetime—and that practicing a martial art three times a week would surely result in a high level of physical fitness.

Pick up any martial arts book and you're likely to read about the physical prowess of martial arts practitioners. You're also likely to run across a much-used (even overused) saying: Practicing a martial art benefits the mind, body, and spirit. We know how the body benefits. And, like the body, the mind is also exercised. Performing different moves with different parts of the body—often at the same time—sharpens the mind by forcing students to concentrate on what they're doing, as opposed to allowing your mind to wander while your body runs through a series of repetitive exercises. Indeed, many women excel at the martial arts because what they lack in strength, they make up for in mental ability.

How the martial arts benefits the spirit is less clear than how the arts benefits the body and the mind. That's because there is greater room for interpretation. What's spiritual to one student isn't to another. In fact, there is such a wide divergence of opinion among students and martial arts masters that it is important to dispel the notion that any person's definition is the "right" one. That applies equally to how martial artists define the mind-body-spirit connection. Just a quick look through several martial arts publications proves this. Consider how the following writers interpret the mind-body-spirit connection:

In his book, *The Spirit of Aikido*, Kisshomaru Ueshiba describes the "three levels of mastery: physical, psychological and spiritual." On the physical level is the kata, he says. On the psychological and spiritual levels, Ueshiba uses time to differentiate between them. He states that psychological ,changes take place from the "very beginning of study," while "the spiritual mastery is inseparable from the psychological but begins only after an intensive and lengthy period of training. . . . Ultimately, physical, psychological, and spiritual mastery are one and the same."

"However you choose to define it, the art of karate has many dimensions: it is at once mental and physical, artistic and grotesque, practical (self-defense) and nonpractical (sport), violent and graceful, abstract and concrete, and scientific and animistic. Irreconcilable contradictions? I don't think so."
The Fundamentals of Goju-Ryu Karate by Gosei Yamaguchi

"The purpose for developing kata also varied with the times and with the people who developed them. For example, in China over 1600 years ago kata was developed and practiced for the purpose of self-defense, whereas the Buddhist monks would practice kata for the purpose of strengthening the spirit as well as the body."
Traditional Karatedo by Morio Higaonna

"Americans, even many martial artists, are accustomed to scoff at tales of the supernatural, the inexplicable, the spiritual. But such is a major aspect of martial arts tradition. And it is not simply a mythology from the past. Even today such events are occurring; and sometimes, though not often discussed, they happen to the most pragmatic, levelheaded, nonmystical martial artists around."
—*Black Belt* magazine, 1983

"In aikido the word ki is used to describe inner power or spirit; and we recognize it as our primary source of energy. . . . Since everything has ki, no simple definition will be adequate. Some of the words that we use in our attempt to define ki are energy, intention, spirit, vital or life force. . . . The body, the mind, and the spirit must be balanced for efficient use or projection of ki."
—*The Essence of Aikido* by Bill Sosa and Bryan Robbins

Where does that leave us with the spiritual side of the martial arts?

At one end of the spirituality spectrum are those martial arts students whose only reward for their hard work is physical. Though they may be aware that there is a spiritual side to the martial arts, they are not interested in exploring it. When the class meditates prior to beginning their physical workouts, for example, these students sit quietly with their eyes closed like the rest of the students, but hardly try to achieve any spiritual level, much less empty their minds of any thoughts, which is what students are expected to do during this exercise. In fact, their minds might be racing. They might be mulling over the day's events. Or maybe they're running through a recently learned kata.

Consider Masutatsu Oyama, a well-known martial artist famous for his flamboyant training techniques, which involve breaking the horns off a live bull (a feat he likes to record through full-color photos in his books). Though he might argue that there is a great deal of spirituality in this feat, many, including myself, would argue otherwise.

At the other end of the spirituality spectrum are those who go beyond the physical to achieve a high degree of spiritual strength. The aikido master described in Chapter 1 is one such person. He uses his chi to plant himself to the ground so firmly that the force of several people pushing him will not cause him to move even an inch. Other chi masters have been known to throw an attacker with a light touch of their hands.

Both types of students—those who choose to ignore the spiritual side of the martial arts and those who embrace it— have chosen to use their minds and strength in different ways. Master Oyama's strength is mainly physical, while the martial artist who plants himself to the ground depends on his spiritual strength, or chi.

Though different in their approaches to the martial arts, these martial artists are similar in that they practice their style to suit themselves. They have interpreted the martial arts in such as way as to fit their beliefs and lifestyles. And therein lies one of the secrets of the martial arts: Though the martial arts demands that students follow the rules and styles of their schools, the martial arts leaves students a great deal of room to individualize their styles.

We've already seen how martial arts instructors interpret styles for their own schools, resulting in styles that are variations on the original founders' visions. For example, katas often get modified by instructors who believe they have found a better way to perform the moves within the katas. This concept applies equally to the spiritual side of the martial arts.

The spiritual side of the martial arts is just another aspect that is open to interpretation. If two students of equal rank climb to the top of a mountain to practice their katas, they may do so for different reasons. One may do it to feel nearer to God; the other because the air is cleaner. Both students are nevertheless martial artists of equal stature.

Most martial arts students probably fall somewhere between being spiritual zealots and uninterested spiritual bystanders. What's more, the student you consider a spiritual martial artist might not think of herself that way. Indeed, ask five students to define the spiritual side of the martial arts, and you're likely to get five different answers.

Ties to Buddhism

As described in Chapter 3, the spiritual aspects of the martial arts grew as the need to protect oneself in the war-torn East diminished. This allowed the arts' religious roots to begin to play a more important role. Today, when students speak of the spiritual nature of the martial arts, very often they are referring to the arts' ties to Buddhism, a religion founded in India in the sixth century B.C. It teaches that right living, right thinking, and self-denial will enable the soul to reach Nirvana, a divine state of release from earthly and bodily pain, sorrow, and desire.

Tied to Buddhism is an offshoot sect known as Zen. It differs from other Buddhist sects in that it seeks enlightenment through introspection and intuition. Its early masters were monks who had become disenchanted by the materialism within Buddhism.

Early Zen masters and the martial artists who tried to follow Zen teachings did not believe that they were training the mind to conform to arbitrary patterns imposed on them by someone else. Rather, they wanted to develop their natural ability to respond to a situation by instinct alone—a concept still very much a part of the martial arts.

Coinciding with the spiritual concepts of Buddhism and

Zen are the concepts of simple, basic living. The martial arts emphasis on continuous repetition of basic moves reflects this tie to these spiritual concepts. Indeed, just as religious leaders chant prayers over and over, martial arts students repeat simple moves again and again.

Also tied to the spiritual concept of simple living is the absence of extraneous paraphernalia in a martial arts school. Certainly, the surroundings inside most schools can be characterized as stark. The walls are often painted white and the floor is bare or covered with a large mat. Very often the only wall hangings are a picture of the style's founder and a list of rules.

Adding to the spirituality of the martial arts is the influence of yoga, which was brought from India to China during the fifth and sixth centuries by Zen Buddhist monks and nuns, who also brought with them Indian fistfighting techniques similar to modern karate. The influences of yoga are still seen in the martial arts breathing techniques and the focus on the inner self.

The prominent role that meditation plays in the martial arts also serves to strengthen the spirituality of the sport. Though meditation has many spiritual connotations, not all of them pertain to every martial arts student. Meditating is a very personal exercise, one that differs for each person doing it. Therefore, there is no right or wrong way to do it. When you feel yourself getting frustrated that you're not meditating correctly or that you can't achieve the peace of mind you think you should, remember this saying attributed to an English abbot, "Meditate as you can, not as you can't." It is a powerful reminder that if you're comfortable meditating and you get something out of it, then you're probably doing it right.

When I meditate with the class, I simply try to erase all thoughts, until my mind is a blank. With my eyes closed, I concentrate until all I "see" is darkness, concentrating the whole time on my breathing. As air is pulled in through my nose, I feel it traveling to my stomach, as my stomach and not my rib cage expands, then up to exit through my mouth. Though not a very deep form of meditation, it relaxes and refreshes me so I can concentrate on class.

Spirit can also be interpreted in an emotional sense, as being in good spirits. Certainly, much has been written about the chemical effects of exercise on the state of a person's mind. Lots of exercise results in high levels of the natural feel-good chemical endorphin. I've often thought that the best part of my martial arts workout was the drive home when I would experience that natural high that comes after your body has been stretched and pushed and the toxins stored up inside you have been sweated out.

How would you interpret the spiritual side of the martial arts? Maybe you feel strongly about finding a school that will allow you to explore this side of the martial arts. Or maybe you're not interested in this aspect. But it is yet another feature to note when choosing schools and observing classes.

But even if you never give the spiritual side of the martial arts a second thought during your training, it won't matter. Just be aware that there is a spiritual side present, and that you can draw on that spiritual strength when physically you feel drained. Mind over matter really does apply in the martial arts. But, again, remember that the spiritual nature of the martial arts is exactly what you make of it.

The Picture of Femininity

In their book *The Martial Arts*, authors Susan Ribner and Dr. Richard Chin feature a picture of a nineteenth-century Japanese woodcut depicting two women fencing with naginatas. From Chapter 1, we know that the naginata is a long pole with a sword set in its end, and was commonly referred to as "the woman's spear."

The women in the picture wear traditional attire: long, flowing kimonos, tight, high black wigs, and makeup. Their calm demeanors, and the absence of any bloodshed implies that they are practicing self-defense moves rather than actually fighting. A third women sits patiently in the background, her hands resting daintily on her lap, as she observes the two women. She is probably waiting for her turn to practice using the naginata.

Though just a simple woodcut, it speaks volumes about women and the martial arts. It clearly states that studying a martial art need not mean abandoning femininity, and in fact, the martial arts can enhance femininity. Certainly, the three women described above, from their attire to their demeanors, are the picture of femininity.

The women could also be twentieth-century role models. Take that woodcut, update it for today's society, and you have an image many advertisers want associated with their products. Indeed, the picture has a lot in common with the way in which modern-day athletic women are depicted in the media. Those print ads from companies selling everything from athletic footwear to bottled water are really just twentieth-century versions of the naginata woodcut.

The Japanese woodcut also depicts women as capable martial arts students, a concept I have tried to convey throughout this book, and one that is shared by many in the martial arts community. In his book *The Spirit of Aikido*, author Kisshomaru Ueshiba writes: "It seems that women generally have more stamina, patience, and the will to continue on the path, and this is probably related to unconscious creative power that they possess. Women who enter the gates of aikido rarely leave training soon after they begin. At least eight out of ten continue, and the longer and deeper they study, the more they become enraptured with aikido."

Finally, the woodcut depicts these three women as having an abundant amount of self-confidence, self-esteem, and composure. Though it could be said that if practiced regularly and passionately enough, any sport will imbue a greater sense of self, it seems even more so when it comes to women in the martial arts. Perhaps it has something to do with the fact that in the martial arts, women and men practice together. Most of us are self-conscious enough in front of women when we attempt to learn something new, but add men to the mix and the possibility for embarrassment goes sky high.

Women who persevere in their training are bound to gain self-confidence, self-esteem, and composure. In *Women in the Martial Arts,* author Carol A. Wiley features the essays of twenty-two women martial artists. Though they all have different stories to tell, the women share the belief that their lives improved through their training.

One such student wrote that she had no direction in her life: no education, no self-esteem, no aspirations. "I experienced many sexual assault attempts by both strangers on the street and guys I knew and trusted. I often wondered if I had a giant bull's eye on me saying, 'Here's a perfect target.'" Her training forced her to challenge herself and change who she was. "A high level of belief in myself has resulted from these changes. Call it self-esteem, self-respect, or self-pride, but it stems from the core of the self," she wrote.

Another student wrote: "I walk with the easy, natural grace of an athlete. My self-confidence is communicated in body language that makes me an unlikely target for hassling."

Wiley herself says self-defense is more a mental attitude than a specific set of techniques. Surely, it's been shown that simply walking with a confident gait deters would-be attackers. But equally important is the benefit you gain of feeling good about yourself. This empowering of the self is probably what kept me coming back to the martial arts throughout my training, but it wasn't always that way.

In my twenties, karate was more of a way for me to channel my energy in a productive way, rather than a way to gain self-confidence. Though I always liked to exercise, I was never into organized sports, and my forays with aerobics classes were disappointing. I also liked the idea that karate classes were held on certain days at specific times. This way I wasn't constantly feeling guilty about not exercising. With karate, I could go to class, then not have to think about working out until the next class.

But if during my twenties the martial arts was something I did mostly to burn calories, by my early thirties, it had become more of a lifestyle than a hobby. Like eating and sleeping, I would feel out of sorts if I didn't get to class two or three times a week.

As I approach my midthirties, I find myself contemplating a return to the martial arts following a hiatus to write this book and give birth to my son. At this point in my life, I can especially appreciate a sport that I began in my early twenties and can return to in my midthirties. Sure, I'll be out of shape compared to the other students, I won't be able to remember all my katas, and I may have passed my physical peak, but it doesn't really matter.

Returning to the martial arts will again mean something different. I'm not going just for a good workout, and I certainly won't be able to give it the prominence in my life that it held before. I see it now as but one small part of an overall healthy lifestyle. That means I won't be able to arrive early to class and stay after class has ended in order to practice my katas. And maybe I'll only be able to get to class once or twice a week. It means making the most of the time I will be able to devote to the martial arts.

Even from just a few hours every week, I'll not only improve my physical appearance, but my mental outlook as well. I'll gain a more positive attitude and a tremendous feeling of accomplishment. For every minute I'll spend sweating and thinking and even cursing the day I ever walked into a martial arts school, I'll gain an inner peace and new insight into my self.

As my life gets more hectic, the martial arts reminds me that you can't rush through something that's important to you. Indeed, studying the martial arts acts as a natural balancing agent to a busy lifestyle.

I'll never regret the day I gathered up the courage to enter a martial arts school and say I'm interested in joining. If every women who ever wanted to take up a martial art actually did, I believe there would be a martial arts school on every corner. Certainly, more and more women continue to join these schools. And, certainly, it's no longer true that the martial arts discourages women from joining. Indeed, a peek inside any school would reveal an albeit small, but healthy contingent of women kicking and punching right alongside their male counterparts.

It is my hope that this book de-mystifies the martial arts to the point where it gives women the courage to seek out the best school and style for them. Armed with the knowledge of what makes for a superior teacher and school, the differences between styles, what they will be expected to learn and what they should expect from their school, walking into a school and saying "I'm interested in joining" becomes that much easier.

Where do you go from here? Well, rather than reread the entire book (although rereading certain sections can be helpful), follow the checklist below. It summarizes how to select a style and school that's right for you.

• Make a list of the styles you think would best suit you. You can start by rereading the style descriptions in Chapter 2. Also, if you know anyone who studies, or has studied, a martial art, ask them why they chose it and what they like about it. (It's fairly easy to find people who started practicing a martial art only to stop after a short while. These people may not have found the right school for themselves, but they can still be great sources of information, so seek out their advice, too.)

• If you're unsure of what style to study, educate yourself on specific styles by reading martial arts magazines and books. There are books on every conceivable martial arts style, and some of these books are even written by women. (*See* Bibliography.)

Or consider a subscription to *Fighting Women News*, an informal quarterly magazine written for women martial artists available only by subscription. It contains articles on martial arts styles, sparring, and self-defense. Subscriptions may be obtained by writing to *Fighting Women News*, Debra L. Pettis, Editor/Publisher, 6741 Tung Avenue West, Theodore, Alabama 36582. Subscribers can obtain a free listing of schools that have women instructors by sending a self-addressed stamped envelope to the above address.

• See how many, if any, schools offer your choice of styles in your area. Your search will probably involve no more than flipping through the yellow pages.

• Once you've narrowed down your choices to the schools you like, call and ask if you can observe a class. Ask to speak with the head instructor. If he is unavailable, try to talk with one of the school's other instructors if there is more than one. Certainly, you're entitled to ask several general questions—What's the average number of students per class? How long do classes run? But don't take up a lot of the instructor's time. There will be plenty of time to ask more questions after observing a class.

• When observing a class, pay particular attention to the instructor. A good instructor gives the class structure, communicates effectively and clearly, maintains control of the class, focuses on students' individual needs, treats students equally, and teaches technique and history and terminology. He also is respected, and returns that respect to his students.

• Then focus on the style. Is it a pure form of the style you've chosen, or a mix of several styles that the instructor has strung together? (If you can't tell by observing the class, ask the instructor afterward.)

• Next, look at the character of the school. Is it loud and noisy? Quiet and focused? Are the floors clean? Is there a trophy case? (If there is, it may indicate that the instructor expects his students to compete in tournaments, or perhaps some of his students just like to compete.)

• Finally, focus on the students. A lot of talking among students before and during class signals a relaxed, less traditional school. Do they take the initiative to work out on their own, or are they milling about waiting for the instructor to begin class? Do they warm up before class? That's a sign of students serious about their art. Do the new students look comfortable and eager? That's a plus, as you may soon be in their shoes.

• If you're interested in the school, ask to take a trial class or two. This will be the true test as to whether you feel the school is right for you.

• Once you've found a school, make sure you purchase the proper uniform. Though hard to detect by an untrained eye, uniforms do differ—even those within the same martial arts style. Ask the instructor what style he requires and where you can purchase it. Double-check with the merchant. Ask him if he knows what uniform is preferred by the instructor in your school. The last thing you want to do is plunk down $80 for a uniform you can't wear or that is different from the others in your class.

• Put off purchasing protective gear until instructed by your teacher. You won't need it until you've mastered some basic moves, and you'll probably want to wear the same type of equipment worn by the rest of the class. In my early training, for example, I would have felt out of place wearing a rib protector because no one else wore one.

• Purchase two comfortable, high-quality sport bras, as well as a couple of new white T-shirts. The bras will make your workout more comfortable. And since most martial arts jackets are loose and open, you'll need a T-shirt to cover yourself. Also, your teacher may instruct the class to work out without their jackets, and you wouldn't want to feel self-conscious about wearing a worn, raggedy T-shirt.

• Make a point of working with every student in your class. You'll become more expert at your moves having performed them with various-size partners.

• Warm-up and stretch out before each class. You'll avoid pulled muscles, and your techniques will look that much smoother.

• Remember, in addition to the mental and spiritual aspects, you're taking up a martial art for fitness and fun, so relax and enjoy yourself.

Bibliography

CLEARY, THOMAS. *The Japanese Art of War.* Boston: Shambhala Publications Inc., 1991.

CORCORAN, JOHN AND EMIL FARKAS. *Martial Arts: Traditions, History, People.* New York: Gallery Books, 1983.

HARRINGTON, PAT. *Judo: A Pictorial Manual.* Tokyo: Charles E. Tuttle Co. Inc, 1992.

HIGAONNA, MORIO. *Traditional Karatedo: Fundamental 1 Techniques.* Tokyo: Kodansha International/USA, Ltd., through Harper & Row, 1985.

HYAMS, JOE. *Zen in the Martial Arts.* Los Angeles: J.P. Tarcher Inc., 1979.

INOSANTO, DAN. *Jeet Kune Do: The Art and Philosophy of Bruce Lee.* Los Angeles: Know Now Publishing Co., 1976.

KIM, RICHARD. *The Weaponless Warriors: An Informal History of Okinawan Karate.* Burbank, Calif.: Ohara Publications Inc., 1974.

MITCHELL, DAVID. *The Martial Arts Coaching Manual.* London: A & C Black Limited, 1988.

MUSASHI, MIYAMOTO. *A Book of Five Rings: The Classic Guide to Strategy.* Woodstock, New York: The Overlook Press, 1974.

OYAMA, MASUTATSU. *The Kyokushin Way: Mas. Oyama's Karate Philosophy.* Tokyo: Japan Publications Inc., 1979.

————*What Is Karate?* Tokyo: Japan Publications Trading Co., 1966.

RANDOM, MICHEL. *The Martial Arts.* London: Octopus Books Limited, 1978.

RIBNER, SUSAN AND DR. RICHARD CHIN. *The Martial Arts.* New York: Harper & Row, Publishers, Inc., 1978.

ROBBINS, BRYAN AND BILL SOSA. *The Essence of Aikido.* Burbank, Calif.: Unique Publications, 1987.

UESHIBA, KISSHOMARU. *The Spirit of Aikido.* Tokyo: Kodansha International Ltd., 1987.

URBAN, PETER. *The Karate Dojo.* Tokyo: Charles E. Tuttle Co. Inc., 1967.

WILEY, CAROL A. *Women in the Martial Arts.* Berkeley, Calif.: North Atlantic Books, 1992.

WILSON, WILLIAM SCOTT. *The Ideals of the Samurai: Writings of Japanese Warriors.* Burbank, Calif.: Ohara Publications Inc., 1982.

YAMAGUCHI, GOSEI. *The Fundamentals of Goju-Ryu Karate.* Los Angeles, Calif.: Ohara Publications, Inc., 1972.